THE DEFEAT *of* COVID

500+ medical studies show what works and what doesn't

April 3, 2021

ISBN: 978-0-578-24821-9 (paperback)
ISBN: 978-0-578-24827-1 (hardback)

Medical Choice Editions

Preface

"There already exist numerous ways to reliably
prevent, mitigate, and even cure COVID-19,
including in late-stage patients
who are already ventilator-dependent."
- Thomas Levy, MD JD

The studies on mask hazards included in this book are the most comprehensive compilation of studies on this topic in the English language. I am honored to have been part of this team project, working with co-authors Boris Borovoy, Maria Crisler and Dr. Q Makeeta on these papers.

If anyone takes first place in my mind as the hero of the COVID-19 era, I think that is Zev Zelenko MD. His treatment success with his own patient population in the epicenter of peak COVID-19 incidence has shown the world what must be done, both for those with this disease and those who are at high risk. For a disease that had once been thought to have a case fatality rate (CFR) of over 3%, in Dr. Zelenko's patients in this study, the CFR was 0.71% with early treatment. That is, only one of 141 patients died in the treatment group, versus 3.5% in the untreated group.[1] This book will examine the mechanisms of why the Zelenko Protocol works so well, and many more studies confirming its success. If this country and the world had heeded what Dr. Zelenko tried to tell us every day during the worst part of the pandemic, there might have been a tremendous number of lives saved. Dr. Zelenko was nominated for the Presidential Medal of Freedom for his outstanding work with COVID-19 patients, and I would go so far as to opine that Dr. Zelenko is deserving of the Nobel Prize in Medicine.

The people I want to thank for inspiring me are those who have shown courage in the face of vicious attacks over the past year of the COVID-19 phenomenon. The following are physicians who disagreed publicly with the pandemic paradigm and were publicly attacked when they offered realistic and practical alternatives to the unmitigated despair promoted by the media and most public figures in government.

Scott Jensen, MD is a practicing physician and a state senator in Minnesota. He did the necessary job that mainstream journalists failed to do. He announced the financial basis of the COVID-19 hysteria in the US, which was the US CARES Act. This unpublicized Act of Congress incentivized COVID-19 diagnoses over influenza and pneumonia. Doctors and hospitals had been told to defer treatment of cancer patients and heart disease patients. Heart disease and cancer are the two biggest killers in the US, each claiming about 600,000 lives per year, and these patients were told their health concerns must be deferred as all attention turned toward the pandemic. Suddenly, hospitals lost their traditional revenue streams, and became COVID-19 hospitals, now with Medicare reimbursement of $13,000 per patient versus only $ 5,000 for flu and pneumonia patients. PCR cycle thresholds for "the COVID-19 test" were raised so high that many people were "testing" positive for COVID-19. Was Dr. Jensen thanked and praised for exposing this deceitful underside of the pandemic phenomenon? No. He was viciously attacked, and his medical board threatened to remove his medical license over his outspokenness.

Medical boards likewise threatened each of the prominent Frontline Doctors for outspoken championing of feasible, well-established and inexpensive medications that had resolved COVID-19 in their patients. Simone Gold MD JD, Richard Urso MD, Stella Immanuel MD, James Todaro MD and Dan Erickson MD are some of the most courageous doctors in the US, and we are extremely lucky to have them as contemporaries, as they provided intelligent, well-reasoned, well-researched and easily followed guidance, in order to emerge from the pandemic. These, America's Frontline Doctors, showed us how to put patient needs first over party-line dogma and dictates from the hierarchy in the pharmaceutical industrial complex that has engulfed other large industries. These doctors dared to prioritize the wellbeing of their patients above dictatorial medicine and showed us how to treat COVID-19. Countless more scientists and physicians and journalists around the world have faced ostracism by their peers when attempting to objectively view and disseminate data regarding COVID-19 and its impacts.

The cover photo of this book shows a nearby cloudy sky, but clearing in the distance. Confusion is rampant among the public in the US and around the world in 2020 – 2021 regarding the phenomenon of COVID-19 and impacts of governments' and media's responses to it. The aim of this book is to clear the confusion, and to show what works contrasted with what does not work, in order to help move humanity forward, away from this multi-dimensional crisis, and into a time where we understand the complexities of the tragedy that the world has suffered and how to avoid such an event again.

Colleen Huber, NMD

THE DEFEAT *of* COVID

Colleen Huber, NMD

CONTENTS

PART I: Pandemic? Mortality & Unpublicized data

PART II: What works: Therapeutics against COVID

PART III: What does not work against COVID

Introduction

Which has had more impact on the world: A coronavirus, or the world's reaction to it? SARS-CoV-2 and COVID-19 have impacted more aspects of human existence than any microbe we have encountered in our lifetimes. Yet, unlike previous pandemics, we have access to plentiful well-tolerated and low-cost treatments with such high rates of success that hospitalization can be minimized or avoided entirely with early treatment. This book will examine those treatments – both how they act, and what impact they have had against COVID-19 in hospitalized patients.

I cite over 500 medical studies in this book. Seven of the chapters have been published already as peer-reviewed articles. The studies cited involve humans, mostly COVID-19 patients with control groups, and seldom animals. Cited studies of mechanisms, or how the treatments actually work, are usually done in laboratory cell cultures. This book is heavily reliant on state-of-the-art immunology and virology for several paragraphs in each chapter. I try to avoid jargon when possible, or to provide definitions when necessary, so that the text can be straightforward and accessible for any reader. The glossary at the end of the text may help. If the reader chooses to skip those technical paragraphs, this book will still provide plenty of resources for the layperson: real world data on each of the treatments in COVID-19 patients around the world. For each of those 500 studies, several more could have been cited, in order to further explore nuanced considerations of the topics presented. But I did not go into that much detail, because I wanted to present a basic overview of the best ways to deal with this pandemic – from the level of the individual and household, all the way to governmental levels, so there should be only enough information here for that purpose, not for all the details and nuances of every tool used for dealing with COVID-19 that may be explored by future researchers. All of the starting points for those considerations may be found in the following chapters.

I also examine the things that don't work against COVID-19. Masks and mask mandates have failed spectacularly against COVID-19. My research team has compiled the most comprehensive research in the English language on the hazards of masks. We found evidence that masks create multiple physiological and microbial imbalances as well as dangerous debris in the body. In addition to those chapters, I explore the blatant irony of masks: Masks made COVID-19 worse in every way. The reader will not only find demographic data showing that mask use was correlated with *higher* rates of COVID-19, but I also show the physics and chemistry of why that happened. As for lockdowns, I proved them to be correlated with more, not fewer, deaths. I cite and link to and screenprint CDC data on that topic.

I have spent my career working with cancer patients as a naturopathic oncologist. Why do I care about COVID-19? First, as a human alive in the western world today, it is impossible not to care about this ubiquitous, multi-faceted phenomenon. Second, I care because the injuries that my research team has discovered about mask hazards will likely lead to many new cases of cancer. If you read this book, you will see evidence that masks injured every organ system that our research team looked at, and that the chronic diseases that masks insidiously begin are known to be much less treatable than is COVID-19. I consider masks to be the worst public health hazard of our time.

Back to the optimistic half of this book, two of the strongest tools against COVID-19 happen to also be two essential tools against cancer, which I have dosed many thousands of times with patients and myself for the last 14 years: Vitamin D and zinc. My clinic has had an equipoise policy for its 14 years of existence. That is, if I ask a patient to take a particular medication or course of treatment, then I should have already taken the same or higher dose myself first, multiple times. I am still waiting, but not holding my breath, for the chemotherapy oncologists to follow my example with their own medicine. In my clinic, I was the first to get in the hyperbaric oxygen chamber, and the first to get various combinations of IV and oral nutrients. As I joke with the patients, "If this kills me, then please don't do it." So the chapters on nutrients will mention doses that I have taken myself, but I am not prescribing for those whom I have never met in clinical consult. For proper individual dosing, a health care consult is advisable with a qualified practitioner.

My patients often ask me for "antiviral herbs" even more so now than before the COVID era. Although botanical medicine has always fascinated me, I have to admit this limitation: The antiviral activity of any herb, even such formidable ones as garlic, boneset and oregano, are probably not going to be quite so effective against COVID-19 as the nutrients and drugs considered herein, so I don't discuss herbs much in this book. For example, the ancient Sumerians, Egyptians, Chinese, Indians, Tibetans, Israelites, Arabs, Greeks and Romans used garlic medicinally.[2] Those whose ancestors survived the bubonic plague (caused by the bacteria *Yersinia pestis*, not viruses) are here to be able to praise the garlic that may have saved those distant ancestors, and thus enabled our existence today.[3 4] But viruses use different mechanisms against their hosts than bacteria.

Even when herbs were able to stop viral replication in laboratories, they usually did not succeed in doing this either in mice or humans. For example, if 12.5% solution of Elderberry in a petri dish can stop viral replication, that is nice, but there is no way that you will get to 12.5% concentration of Elderberry in your blood. So human *in vivo* trials of herbs vs SARS-CoV-2 have not had as much measurable effect as *in vitro* studies of viral inactivation. What herbs *can* do is to stimulate immune function, and this is what we want to accomplish with them. For example, even potent garlic's "antiviral" effect is likely more due to its impact on immune function.[5] Although there are many herbs throughout the world long valued for this purpose, they have not yet been observed to match the impact of the nutrients and drugs discussed herein, specifically in their ability to stimulate immune function against COVID-19.

Antiviral is a misleading word, because in the case of nutrients it refers to two distinct steps in a process, rather than one. Treatment → immune enhancement → viral inactivation = "antiviral" treatment. In this book, I use the word *antiviral* to mean the effects on the human immune system that in turn stop viral replication or viral entry into cells or other tasks that are accomplished by the innate and adaptive immune system. In the case of the two drugs discussed in this book, hydroxychloroquine and ivermectin, the virucidal effect against SARS-CoV-2 is more direct against the virus. In the case of the nutrients discussed, their primary value by far is the strengthening of the immune system.

Optimal time for treatment of COVID-19 has been found to be early in the infectious process, at the time of infection and during the incubation period, before infection spreads from the upper to the lower respiratory tract, and before severe inflammation begins.[6] But that is not the only time, and each treatment discussed herein has also shown impressive, often life-saving, effect in gravely ill COVID-19 patients.

As I will show throughout this book, the virus SARS-CoV-2 and the disease known as COVID-19 don't stand a chance against vitamin D or zinc or vitamin C or hydroxychloroquine or ivermectin.

It would be difficult if not impossible for a person not already hospitalized from different diseases to die of COVID-19, with an adequate amount of any of these, and especially if using a well-chosen combination of them.

This book is as much about treatment as prevention. We have learned from worldwide clinical trials that ivermectin is so powerful against COVID-19 that one study showed greater impact on survival of critically ill COVID-19 patients than on early stage patients.[7] The chapter on ivermectin shows tremendous effect on clinical trials and the extraordinarily advantageous mechanisms of this 36 year old medicine against SARS-CoV-2, locking and blocking its activity beautifully at all key steps.

COVID-19 and COVID are used almost interchangeably throughout this book, as variants have emerged, which take COVID past its 2019 beginning. The former refers to specific findings of clinical studies, and is used in the seven peer-reviewed studies that comprise seven chapters of this book. The second refers to the entire COVID phenomenon as an evolving virus as well as the new historical era we are living through.

An essential topic to consider regarding the COVID-19 phenomenon is the mRNA injections being incorrectly called "vaccines." This topic is the most heavily fraught with financially and politically driven agendas and censorship. When pursued honestly, science, as it always must, rises above such considerations. However, at this writing the COVID injections are only a few months into their widespread use in the general public. Much speculation has abounded, and real data is still wanting. One year, five years from now, we will know so much about what these vaccines did, that anything I write now will be quickly outdated. For example, will these mRNA injections have similar outcomes to those used for dengue fever in the Philippines? Will the cationic lipid coating be problematic? How shall we compare adverse events after the mRNA injections with adverse events associated with

COVID-19? I believe it is too early to give credible answers to these questions.

The most important consideration regarding any vaccine is addressed in the pages of this book, but not from the usual perspective of "pro" or "anti." From Jenner's earliest experiments with cowpox to the latest technology with mRNA delivery, all vaccines have one thing in common: They stimulate B cells to produce antibodies, and that is their sole recognized and reliable immune function, although farther immune system reach has been a goal occasionally achieved in vaccine development.[8] [9] [10] But B cell function and the antibodies they produce comprise only a tiny part of the entire human immune system. And natural encounter with a pathogenic virus engages the entire immune system. There are about 37 trillion cells in the human body. Each of us has 3 billion B cells (the ones that make antibodies), but we have 300 billion T cells, and that is only the adaptive immune system. The innate immune system has an even much greater diversity and range or ubiquitous presence than the adaptive immune system. Our entire body, every cell in it, is less than a fingernail's thickness away from the nearest blood vessel, and if any cell were further away than that from the bloodstream, it would die. That's how close every bit of the body is to the innate immune system. So the domain of vaccines (any vaccine) in human immune function is quite small compared to total human immune function, and we are at all times, primarily reliant on the rest of the immune system, not on the part that is affected by vaccines.

As we shall see in the following pages, Vitamin D and zinc are ubiquitous in their presence throughout the immune system. These two nutrients have been found to be active – in a pro-human and anti-viral way – everywhere that researchers have looked. Receptors for each have been found in each immune cell studied. If vaccines only act on the B cell/antibody portion of the adaptive immune portion of the human immune system, then Vitamin D and zinc act on *all of it*: The innate immune system, including monocytes, macrophages, mast cells, neutrophils, complement, natural killer cells, dendritic cells and other antigen-presenting cells, as well as the adaptive immune system: not only B cells, but helper T-cells and cytotoxic T-cells. If after reading this book, you meet anyone who thinks a vaccine can be superior to nutrients in defeating infectious diseases, you have met someone who does not know much about immunology or viral infections, or who only cares about less than 1% of immune function.

This book has the date April 3, 2021. Why did I write the date that I finished my book? Because my peer-reviewed published article, "Masks are neither effective nor safe: A summary of the science," has already been stolen by three different parties that I know of, without acknowledging that it was my work. This was not the first time my work has been plagiarized, so I prefer to make it more difficult for it to happen the next time.

My family stopped at a scenic lookout on the Pan American highway a few years ago, and I took some photos of the sunset, and now use one as the cover of this book. The foreground is cloudy, but there are clearer skies in the distance. Although the COVID-19 phenomenon (microbial, physiological, medical, environmental, political, economic, social and cultural) still has many people in the throes of fear, unemployment, isolation, confusion, depression and despair, the goal of this book is to provide clarity and insight toward resolving the current situation, to plan adequate nutritional interventions for future viral infections and outbreaks, and to help prevent a devastating pandemic phenomenon from ever happening again. By the end of this book, the reader may find that there are readily available tools against the ascendance of any future pathogen to the level of a pandemic.

Part I: Pandemic? Mortality and unpublicized data

PDMJ

Data that disprove the COVID-19 pandemic

December 19, 2020.
Completed peer-review and revised, January 18, 2021

https://pdmj.org/papers/is_there_a_pandemic/

Colleen Huber,[i]
Boris Borovoy [ii]

Abstract

A pandemic that calls the attention of the public, and action by the medical field, is one that raises the total death rate above that of a typical year or season. The COVID-19 era that began in early 2020 has received continuous and rapt attention in the United States for deaths that have occurred. Has COVID-19 resulted in more deaths (known as "excess deaths") than would have happened in a typical year? An

---

[i] Colleen Huber, NMD is a Naturopathic Medical Doctor and Naturopathic Oncologist (FNORI), writing on topics of masks, COVID-19, cancer and nutrition.

[ii] Boris A Borovoy, MPH has a Master in Public Health from Moscow Medical Academy.

obstacle to answering that question is that COVID-19 testing is flawed and imprecise, for reasons discussed herein, and it is difficult to distinguish COVID-19 from other respiratory illnesses, due to symptoms and signs that are mostly indistinguishable from the common cold, flu or pneumonia. It is possible that deaths of multiple causes have been ascribed to COVID-19, especially due to new peculiarities in mortality reporting during 2020 discussed herein. Therefore, year-over-year comparison of deaths from all causes is likely the best analysis of available evidence of whether the United States is now confronted by a deadly pandemic. The CDC mortality numbers are as yet unaudited by independent parties. Therefore, we compare numbers of obituaries in 2020 and 2019, which are verifiable reports of deaths of specific, identified individuals. We also examine the earnings statements of the largest medical suppliers in the US, to see if their sales of medical oxygen and other medical equipment prove a pandemic. These data all indicate that there has been no pandemic in the US in 2020.

Background

A pandemic is the prevalent spread of a disease over an entire country or worldwide, and there is often increased mortality for its duration compared to more typical years. Early rises in death rate are a warning of an especially dangerous pandemic. In 2020, it has been widely assumed that COVID-19 is an unusually deadly pandemic.

Understanding the COVID-19 phenomenon has been obstructed by several factors.

COVID-19 is assumed to be caused by a coronavirus that is said to be novel, "SARS-Cov-2." However, SARS is likely a misnomer, because it is an abbreviation of Severe Acute Respiratory Syndrome. It is not at all clear that a majority or even a significant minority of COVID-19 patients have had acute respiratory distress with this illness. Other factors, such as use of over-pressurized ventilators, have led to acute respiratory distress among COVID-19 patients.

The most confusing aspect of COVID-19 is reliance on a manufacturing technique, now nearly universally re-purposed as a test for the presence of the SARS-Cov-2 virus, although there are many problems with this "test." We list these problems below:

1. The very questionable applicability of the manufacturing technique, the reverse-transcriptase / polymerase chain reaction technique for propagating RNA, now used throughout the world as a test for presence of the particular infectious agent in question, or of other coronaviruses, virions and virus particles that may resemble or share common nucleic acid sequences with the SARS-Cov-2 infectious agent, without distinction among those; and
2. The 80% and higher false positive rate of this "test" in the diagnosis of COVID-19, partially due to cross-immunity to fragments of other coronaviruses, inevitably present in the

human body,[11] [12] followed by political pressure to recant these findings; and

3. The arbitrary number of iterations of this "test" (cycle thresholds) that must be selected to produce a positive "result"; and
4. Instructions given to physicians by the CDC to code cases as COVID-19 deaths including presumptively, even though multiple severe co-morbidities are typical among individuals whose deaths were called COVID-19; [13] and
5. Controversy regarding higher Medicare and private insurance reimbursement for COVID-19 patients than for flu patients,[14] [15] which may have skewed reported cause of death on death certificates; and
6. Generous financial rewards to hospitals by the US CARES Act for the number of COVID-19 patients they treat;[16] and
7. The possibility that there may be political influences in altering the true number of deaths from COVID-19.

Two of these problems in particular merit greater attention.

COVID-19 has been very heavily marketed as a pandemic to the US public, with two important aspects that led to false reporting of US mortality data for COVID-19.

The incentive for mis-stated US mortality data is the financial influence created by the US CARES Act, which budgeted $175 billion dollars for distribution to hospitals for treatment of COVID-19 patients, with many hospitals receiving millions of dollars in such aid.[17] Specific financial incentives that favored COVID-19 diagnosis over other similar diagnoses such as flu, pneumonia and bronchitis especially, included a Medicare incentive of only $5,000 per patient for pneumonia, but $13,000 per patient for the pathologically indistinguishable COVID-19 pneumonia.[18] Further, the CARES Act incentive of $39,000 to treat such a patient with a ventilator resulted in financially lucrative outcomes for hospitals, but medically lethal outcomes for patients.[19]

The core of public confusion and fear of COVID-19 stems from the testing itself. Reverse-transcriptase, polymerase chain reaction (RT-PCR) is a manufacturing technique for producing more RNA nucleic acid sequences. It was not intended by its inventor, the late Kary Mullis, PhD, as a test for an infectious disease. He warned against its use in such an application. He especially warned that it could be misused if the cycles, or iterations, of this procedure were processed too many times on a particular specimen. Regarding the use of RT-PCR to attempt to detect infectious disease, he said, at 35 or 40 cycles, "you can find almost anything in anybody."[20] The CDC acknowledges that 33 cycles or more are unlikely to detect active virus.[21] The number of cycles used in "COVID-19 testing" in the US have been above 37, and often well into the 40's for all of 2020.[22] [23] Laboratories in the US do not disclose the cycle thresholds that they use in running RT-PCR SARS-CoV-2 tests, except in Florida where the disclosure is mandatory.[24] No standardization for cycle threshold values exists across different tests and different laboratories.[25]

Infectivity was found to be significantly reduced from positive tests when cycles were greater than 24, and that for every 1-unit increase in cycle threshold, the odds ratio of infectivity decreased by 32%.[26] Researchers concluded that PCR sensitivity is excellent (can find viral particles very easily), but that its specificity for detecting replicative (active) virus is poor,[27] as Dr. Mullis had warned. Nevertheless, RT-PCR has become "the COVID-19 test" used ubiquitously throughout the US and many other countries.

The magnitude of deception resulting from this misuse, overuse, over-cycling and over-advertising of PCR as a COVID-19 testing technique, along with frequent exhortations by politicians to "get tested," can hardly be overstated. This is the core of the problem of the public falsely believing that there is a pandemic, and that its name is COVID-19.

Therefore, in order to attain the truest picture of the impact of the COVID-19 on public health, it would be helpful to look at deaths from all causes, to see if there has been a significant change.

Deaths attributed to COVID-19 are at the oldest ages; yet age distribution of all-cause mortality did not significantly change during weeks of peak reported COVID-19 deaths

Researcher Genevieve Briand PhD hypothesized that the over-counting of COVID-19 death numbers may be due to society's heavy focus on that topic, which would eclipse awareness or even reporting of more typical causes of death.[28]

Dr. Briand found that the proportion of total deaths in US by age group did not change from before COVID-19 to after its peak incidence in the US. The CDC has shown throughout 2020 that peak incidence of COVID-19 deaths occurred the weeks ending April 11 and April 18, 2020,[29] as shown in this graph:

Graph 1

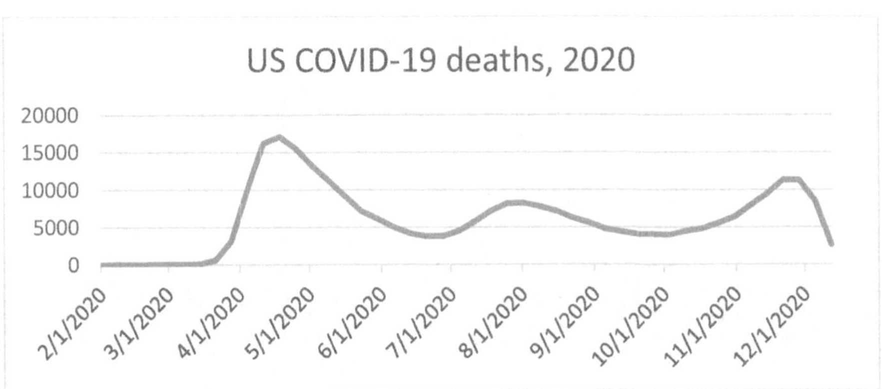

Briand's research showed that for all weeks of 2020 to date, a consistent proportion, among different age groups, of deaths from all causes occurred. Her research was quickly removed from the internet almost as soon as it was posted. The publisher, then censor, was Johns Hopkins University, with known financial ties to World Economic Forum and Bill and Melinda Gates Foundation, each of which has taken an active role in promoting COVID-19 as the catalyst that justifies a New World Order.[30] Several concerns regarding over-reporting of COVID-19 data are enumerated above.

This is Dr. Briand's graph of the age distribution of total deaths from February 1, 2020, which is before COVID-19 affected the US population, before there was even one death from it, through early September 2020.

Graph by Genevieve Briand

Graph 3: Percentage of U.S. Deaths per Age Group, from MMWR week ending 2/1/2020 to week ending 11/14/2020

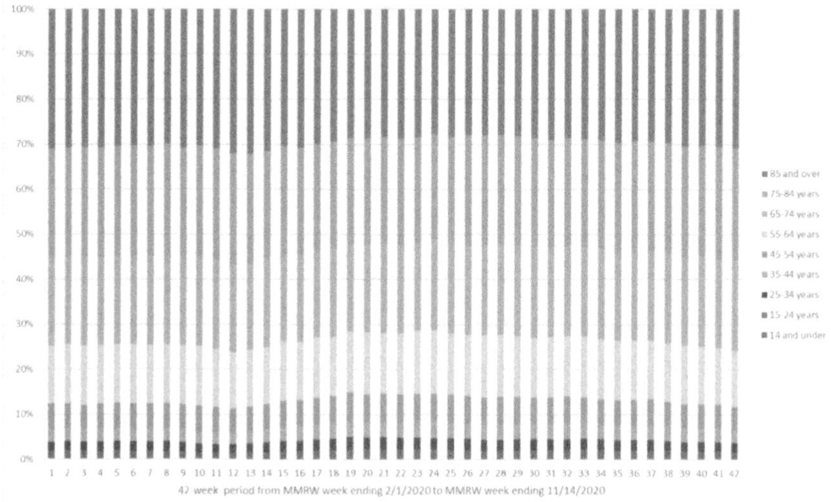

Source: Page 2 of 2 of "Provisional Death Counts for Coronavirus Disease 2019 (COVID-19) By Week of Death" table, https://www.cdc.gov/nchs/nvss/vsrr/covid_weekly/index.htm. Downloaded 12-26-20.

And zoomed in, an earlier version:

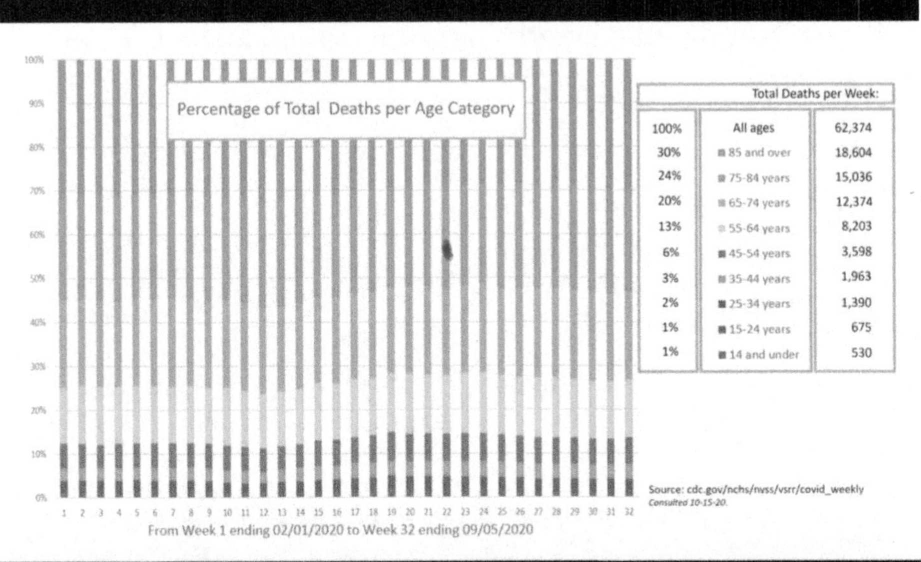

Our updated graph, derived from CDC data through 01/02/2021 [31] of the same analysis is as follows:

Graph 2

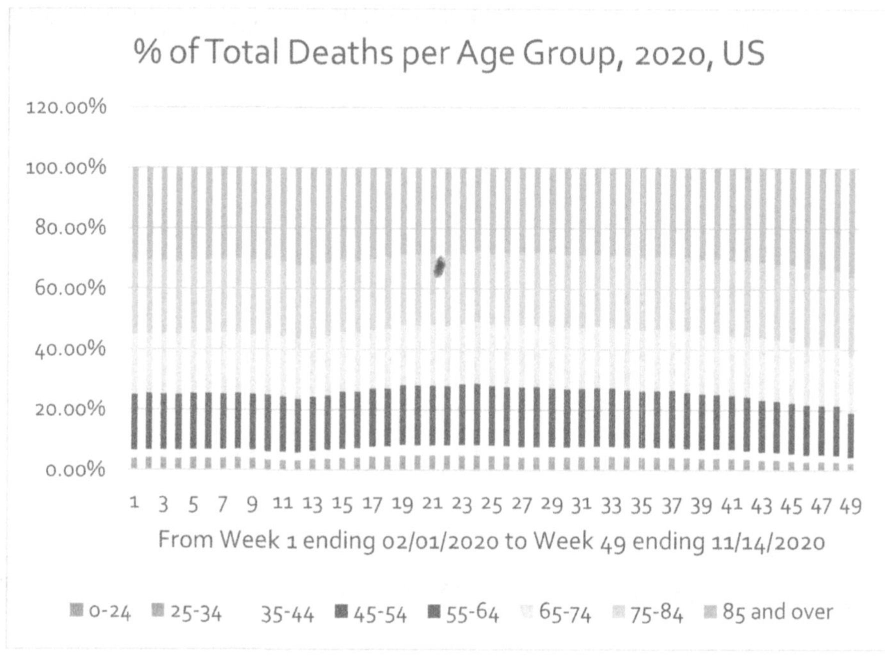

What is especially interesting about the age distribution of total deaths is that there is no extreme change at any time in 2020 of the proportion of total deaths for any age group, except for the last seven weeks, but those weeks do not correspond to COVID-19 peak mortality reporting, which was in April 2020. The CDC showed the weeks ending April 11 and April 18, 2020 (weeks 11 and 12 of the above graph) as the weeks with the highest COVID-19 deaths, yet there is barely perceptible difference in age distribution of deaths, even during those weeks. If there were a pandemic that affected all age groups equally, such a consistency over the year would not be surprising.

However, COVID-19 is a peculiar phenomenon in that the average age of death for COVID-19 is beyond the average age of total deaths.

Unfortunately, regarding COVID-19, much of the important data still remains hidden. The BBC reports average age of death in Scotland is 79.1, but the average age of COVID-19 death in Scotland is 81.5.[32] The mean age of COVID-19 death in France is 79 years.[33] If there were a large number of deaths from COVID-19, with average age of death of 79 to 81, there would have been wide swings in age distribution toward the higher age groups during peak time periods of deaths that were attributed to COVID-19. In comparison with the first four weeks studied (February 2020), when there were no COVID-19 deaths, there would have been a rise in the proportion of those in the highest age categories of all deaths. However, that change did not happen. As Briand concluded, COVID-19 had no effect on the percentage of deaths of older people as a portion of the whole population.

Despite unreliable data resulting from reported PCR positive "cases," much of the world has come to accept a commonly agreed upon Infection Fatality Rate (IFR) for COVID-19. That had been agreed to be 0.26% until March 2021, when it was then pinpointed to IFR = 0.15%, and that approximately 1/4 of the world's population had been infected.[34]

The graph below, from Science,[35] shows age distribution for the Infection Fatality Rate of COVID-19. We see that the deaths are skewed strongly toward the upper ages.

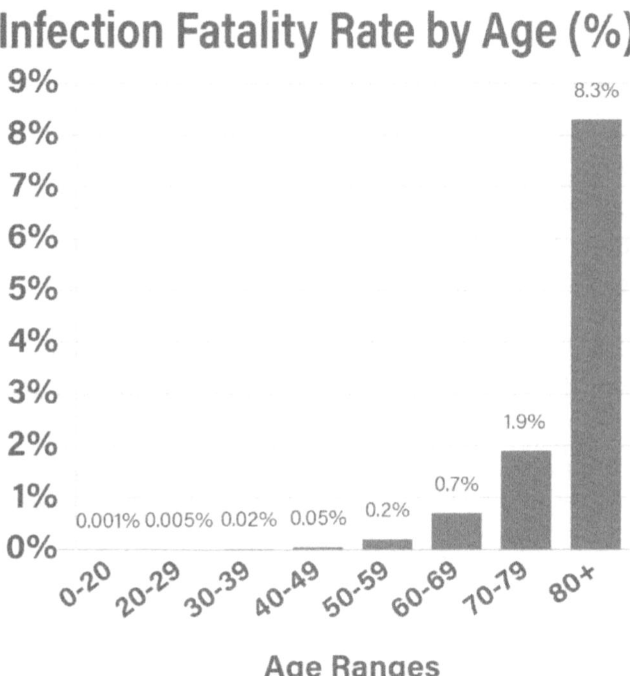

Source: Science 10 Jul 2020;, Vol. 369, Issue 6500, pp. 208-211 DOI: 10.1126/science.abc3517

The average life expectancy in the US is 78.7 to 78.9 years. [36] [37] If the average age of death from COVID-19 is above the average US life expectancy, then COVID-19 cannot be a major independent cause of death, as in cutting short the lives of people who were expected to live longer. This of course varies with individuals, but cannot vary with respect to the population as a whole.

Even from unaudited CDC data so far, it appears that COVID-19 has not made appreciable impact on the overall US death rate. From 2017 through 2020 the rate of deaths in the US population has stayed at 0.9%, keeping pace with population growth, as the following table shows. [38]

DEATHS IN US BY YEAR

Year	Deaths	Population	Deaths per 100,000	Rate
2010	2,468,435	309,346,863	798	0.8%
2011	2,515,458	311,718,847	807	0.8%
2012	2,543,279	314,102,623	810	0.8%
2013	2,596,993	316,427,395	821	0.8%
2014	2,626,418	318,907,401	824	0.8%
2015	2,712,630	321,418,820	844	0.8%
2016	2,744,248	323,071,342	849	0.8%
2017	2,813,503	325,147,121	865	0.9%
2018	2,839,205	327,167,439	868	0.9%
2019	2,855,000	328,239,523	870	0.9%
2020	2,902,664	330,767,888	878	0.9%

CDC - Census (as of 12/30/2020)
https://www.cdc.gov/nchs/nvss/vsrr/provisional-tables.htm
https://www.cdc.gov/nchs/nvss/vsrr/covid19/index.htm

(Numbers reflect all deaths, including Covid-19)

Obituary data

To understand the discrepancy between the announcement of a pandemic that affects almost entirely the elderly, yet does not change the deceased elderly as a proportion of the total deceased, we must look beyond this particular set of data.

The CDC has presented on faith their enumerated death counts. One might ask, but where is the evidence underlying these numbers? Of the largest obituary reporting services in the US, the largest of these with the most transparent data seems to be United States Obituary Notices (USObit.com.) This obituary reporting service reports the deaths of specific, verifiable deceased individuals. The total numbers of deceased reported by USOBit.com are approximately 20% to 25% of total deaths in the US as reported by the CDC. The data shown on their site for 2019 and 2020 is summarized as follows.

Table 1: 2020

Usobit.com US obituary notices	Pages of obituaries	x 12 per page	Total deaths per month	Rank
Jan-20	4772	12	57264	1
Feb-20	4021	12	48252	3
Mar-20	3436	12	41232	10
Apr-20	3850	12	46200	6
May-20	3294	12	39528	12
Jun-20	4182	12	50184	2
Jul-20	3952	12	47424	4
Aug-20	3796	12	45552	7
Sep-20	3444	12	41328	9
Oct-20	3657	12	43884	8
Nov-20	3386	12	40632	11
Dec-20	3885	12	46620	5
Total US deaths accounted for by obituaries - 2020			548100	

Table 1: 2019

Usobit.com US obituary notices	Pages of obituaries	x 12 per page	Total deaths per month
Jan-19	7167	12	86004
Feb-19	5657	12	67884
Mar-19	5293	12	63516
Apr-19	4632	12	55584
May-19	3478	12	41736
Jun-19	4041	12	48492
Jul-19	4066	12	48792
Aug-19	3920	12	47040
Sep-19	4266	12	51192
Oct-19	4289	12	51468
Nov-19	4179	12	50148
Dec-19	4693	12	56316
Total US deaths accounted for by obituaries - 2019			668172

Obituaries of real, identifiable deceased individuals declined by almost 18% from 2019 to 2020. If these obituaries are representative of deaths in the US as a whole, then it is impossible for there to be a pandemic in the United States in 2020. These deaths are at least verifiable, unlike the unaudited, unverified numbers that the CDC presents. It is also interesting that the month with the largest number of COVID-19 deaths according to the CDC, April 2020, ranks 6th out of the 12 months of 2020 regarding total obituaries. Other large obituary services did not respond to requests for information or refused to share information on total numbers of obituaries in 2019 and in 2020.

Wall Street vs the pandemic story

There are other data that suggest that there is no pandemic, at least not involving a pathogen that causes acute respiratory distress.

We looked at companies that produce and distribute medical oxygen. The following graph shows total sales over the largest of those companies actually declined from 2019 to 2020.

Table 2

Company name	NYSE symbol	SALES $ Millions	2017	2018	2019	2020	Half-year revenue 2019 Q1Q2	2019 Q3Q4	2020 Q1Q2
MED O2 PRODUCERS									
Air Products	APD		8188	8930	8919	8857			
Air Liquide	AIQUY						12360	12297	11540
Linde	LIN		11400	14800	28200	27000			
Total sales $M			19588	23730	37119	35857			
Change in medical O2 sales in 2020 from 2019						-3.40%			-6.16%
O2 CONCENTRATOR PRODUCERS									
Invacare	IVC		966.5	972.3	928	842.2			
Inogen	INGN		249.4	358.1	361.9	303.7			
Medtronic	MDT			30000	30600	28900			
Philips	PHG		20100	21400	21800	23700			
ResMed	RMD			2300	2600	3000			
Vapotherm	VAPO		35.6	42.4	48.1	117.1			
Total sales $M				55072.8	56338	56863			
Change in O2 concentrator over previous year					2.30%	0.93%			

At the beginning of 2020, COVID-19 had no perceptible impact on any aspect of life or business in the US. By the end of 2020, almost every facet of American life had been shaken by the phenomenon of the response to SARS-CoV-2. That is, every aspect *except* the public's need for medical oxygen. For the alleged "Severe Acute Respiratory Syndrome" for which SARS-CoV-2 was named, US citizens have actually consumed less supplemental medical oxygen in 2020 than in 2019, despite our growing population, thus disproving a 2020 pandemic involving a respiratory pathogenic virus, i.e. the now legendary SARS-CoV-2 and COVID-19.[39]

In a related market, oxygen concentrators have been recently innovated to include small, portable backpack units for individuals who are ambulatory with long-term chronic conditions requiring supplemental oxygen, which is thought to account for much of the increase in sales in 2019. This welcome innovation greatly increased mobility and convenience for those dependent on supplemental oxygen. But even those sales did not increase as much in 2020 as they had in 2019, and are mostly irrelevant to a virus thought to be as acutely sickening as SARS-CoV-2. Rather, small travel-size backpacks of oxygen concentrators are more suited to ambulatory patients with chronic COPD, pulmonary fibrosis, and other non-emergent lung diseases.

Then we looked at other medical products.

The five largest medical supply companies in the US are: McKesson, Amerisource Bergen, Henry Schein, Cardinal Health and Medline Industries.[40] Their sales for 2019 and 2020, from their corporate earnings reports[41] are compared below, as well as their change in growth over that time.

Table 3

5 largest medical suppliers		SALES in $ Millions						
		2019	2020			Growth rate		
						1 Yr	3 Yr	5 Yr
McKesson		214000	231000			5.50%	5.20%	5.20%
Amerisource Bergen		179500	189900			5.70%	7.40%	6.90%
Henry Schein		10000	9800			-1.70%	-4.80%	-0.80%
Cardinal Health		145500	152900			4.70%	5.60%	8.30%
Medline Industries	not on NYSE							
Total sales		**549000**	**583600**		**Total growth**	**14.20%**	**13.40%**	**19.60%**

Although these five companies' sales increased in 2020 over 2019, the growth rate for one year has slowed from the 5-year aggregate overall growth rate for these companies. This is even though the US population has steadily increased through those years.

Conclusion

On examination of diverse data, from CDC mortality data, to obituaries, to Wall Street earnings reports, there are enough indicators that a pandemic involving a Severe Acute Respiratory Syndrome (SARS) virus could not have taken place, at least not in the United States in 2020.

Part II: What works: Therapeutics against COVID

It is certainly possible and may turn out to be most productive against COVID-19 to use the treatments discussed in this section in combination. For example, I will summarize research that shows that hydroxychloroquine acts to block the entry of SARS-CoV-2 into host cells. Also ivermectin enhances antiviral activity by blocking entry to the cell nucleus, and by inhibiting viral replication. Therefore, a synergy of these decades' old drugs, with long-term safe use in the same populations over that time, may synergize for even stronger effect against SARS-CoV-2 than each has alone. There are no known adverse drug interactions between them.[42]

There is no combination of prevention or treatment regimen against COVID-19 or any other pathogen that excludes the function of vitamin D. Vitamin D is essential to life and to the functioning of the entire immune system, both innate and adaptive; there is no known immune component that has been observed, in laboratory findings, to function uninfluenced by vitamin D. We shall see that nearly as strong arguments may be made for vitamin C and zinc versus COVID-19.

Is COVID another name for deficiency of vitamin D?

"Vitamin D is the bedrock foundation of immunity. It's almost as if vitamin D were designed for COVID."

-- Paul Bergner

Introduction

Is it possible to die from COVID-19 while maintaining adequate serum levels of Vitamin D? COVID-19 is attributed to infection with SARS-CoV-2 coronavirus. SARS, or Severe Acute Respiratory Distress Syndrome is a known risk of vitamin D deficiency, and has been reversed and eliminated by supplementation of the same. Population studies and studies of hospitalized patients with COVID-19 diagnosis show strongly improved outcomes with higher serum levels of vitamin D. Unlike vaccination, which acts on a small portion of immune function, vitamin D receptors are ubiquitous throughout the entire immune system. There is no cell line where vitamin D receptors have been determined to be absent. Vitamin D activates all known immune system functions, and thwarts viral pathogenesis at each step that has been studied. But vitamin D is also essential in stopping some of the most severe over-reactions of the immune system to viral invasion, such as cytokine storm. Is it possible that COVID-19 is another name for deficiency of vitamin D?

Is there a species that has ever existed that was without macroscopic and microscopic predators? In the animal kingdom, we can use our five senses and our wits to detect, evade and escape or chase away our macroscopic predators. The task is more challenging with microscopic predators, normally thought of as pathogenic microbes. Because our senses are not very useful in awareness of either microbial presence nor of our vulnerability to the same, there are different defenses employed by animals, plants and even microbes against pathogenic microbes.

The next three chapters examine the series of events that occurs when the number of virions in the body rises, specifically the human immune response to SARS-CoV-2, the infectious agent in COVID-19, considering both the role of this respiratory virus and the body's response to it.

It has been found, in clinical studies throughout the world, that Vitamin D has a role in every known aspect of human immune function. Discussion of human immune response to this or any other pathogen, without a consideration of the ubiquitous role of Vitamin D, is therefore necessarily incomplete. To give an example of a different intervention, vaccines stimulate antibodies, which are an aspect of the adaptive immune response to pathogenic assault. Vaccines therefore are active in a portion of total immune function, but Vitamin D is active in all human immune functions, as will be shown throughout the next three chapters.

A number of variants have been observed to SARS-CoV-2, all with one or another variation in the spike protein. However, as of this writing, even with widespread findings of variants, "cases," (even with the problematic and highly malleable contemporary definition of a case), hospitalizations and deaths from COVID-19 have dropped precipitously around the world since early January, 2021, prior to widespread vaccination, and including in areas where these variants originated. Therefore, in this chapter we are not concerned with variants of SARS-CoV-2.

The Innate Immune System vs COVID-19

Innate immunity is common throughout the animal kingdom, and 99% of the animal kingdom relies only on the innate system, not having an equivalent to the human adaptive immune system. Epithelial barriers, both skin and mucosa, are the first line of defense. As such, the most expendable skin, the metabolically inactive keratinocytes, are a shield against pathogens, so long as the epidermis is not pierced. When the skin is lacerated, abraded, punctured or otherwise compromised, innate immunity is the organism's first response. Gathering of leukocytes and plasma-borne proteins comprise the early inflammatory process. In the case of cells that have been infected by viruses, those cells are killed by natural killer cells. Type I interferons stop viral replication in infected cells. The amnesic role of the innate immune system is that all pathogens of the same type are treated identically whether similar pathogens have invaded previously or not. It is only later that the adaptive immune system, particularly memory cells, will respond in a more precisely targeted way.

COVID-19 is observed to have an incubation period of 5 days, and if hospitalization occurs, it generally happens within the following 7 days.[43] 80% of the patients who develop symptoms generally get better on their own. The human immune system has been key to this success of this majority. The innate immune system is almost exclusively used in early childhood, and gradually weakens with age, while the importance and capability of, and reliance on, the adaptive immune system increases with age to the point of near exclusive reliance on adaptive immunity in the elderly. It has been observed that innate immune response has been key to successful outcome against COVID-19,[44] which may account for the strong age differential of this disease, of which the average age of death is 81, and children are unaffected.[45]

Fever is one of the early symptoms of COVID-19, if the body is capable of mounting a robust fever. It has been found that fever of 39 degrees Celsius stimulates production in the lymphocytes of more than 10-fold interferon gamma than cells in the same individuals at normal basal temperature.[46] The importance of interferons in the body's fight against viruses can hardly be overstated.

The innate system is the first-responding activity of the immune system. In the innate immune system interferons are the best understood and likely most devastating cytokine produced against viruses. All of our cells have Type I interferons, knows as interferon alpha and interferon beta, which are the first to be activated in the event of a new infection.

SARS-CoV-2 virus has been found to interfere with the body's production of interferon. This is a mechanism of how the virus advances through the immune system. But later when the virus has actively replicated, it has been found that "active viral replication later results in hyper-production of type I interferon and influx of neutrophils and macrophages, which are the major source of inflammatory cytokines." The authors concluded that a pathogenic mechanism of SARS-CoV-2 is that it "probably induces delayed Type I interferons and loss of viral control in an early phase of infection."[47] Or that is, the patients who were found to succumb to the most severe disease outcomes were those that could not produce an early immune response against the virus, particularly those with low Type I interferon activity, as measured by Type I interferon activity and presence in the blood.[48] Patients with auto-antibodies against Type I interferons all had low or undetectable interferons and had severe or life-threatening COVID-19, and none of them had mild cases.[49]

Because of the 10-fold increase in interferon production at a body temperature of 39 degrees Celsius as discussed above, it may be useful to think of strategies to enhance this mechanism. Anti-pyretic medications may be avoided during this time. The naturopathic medical curriculum has for over a century incorporated constitutional hydrotherapy along with the contemporary medical curriculum as well as other traditionally naturopathic fields, such as botanical medicine and nutrition. Practitioners have used successive applications of hot and cold, and or sauna or infrared strategies to induce higher temperature in their patients under controlled conditions to avoid burns.[50]

Vitamin D and the human immune system generally

Vitamin D has been known for a century to be essential to human immune function against pathogenic microbes.[51]

Vitamin D is capable of entering not only the cell but the nucleus as well, and can affect transcriptional change, including to the point of interfering with viral replication. Vitamin D is known to interfere with transcription of viral RNA. Vitamin D is not entirely made within the body, yet it is required for adequate production of many of the body's hormones. So it is a vitamin, by definition, because the body needs it in order to survive.

Vitamin D deficiency is common in autoimmune patients.[52] Vitamin D has an essential role in immune regulation,[53] and has been preventive to helpful to even curative in some of the most common and serious auto-immune diseases, such as inflammatory bowel disease (IBD)[54] and even Type 1 diabetes,[55] and rheumatoid arthritis, where 100% of the RA-induced mice were cured after administration of vitamin D.[56] Immune dysregulation and chronic inflammation are characteristic of the above conditions, and Vitamin D seems to re-regulate the immune system and suppress inflammation, by decreasing NF kappa B, [57] [58] [59] [60] which in turn decreases pro-inflammatory cytokines.[61] Vitamin D was also shown to improve immune tolerance of transplanted organs.[62] Vitamin D cured a polio condition in 100% of laboratory mice. In mice infected with a polio condition, autoimmune encephalomyelitis (AE), 100% showed evidence of AE, which is one of the many synonyms of polio, as the polio virus has not yet been isolated. The researchers mentioned the AE connection with multiple sclerosis, another disease of vitamin D deficiency.[63] [64] In their study, after supplementing 1,25-dihydroxy D3, zero percent of those mice showed AE at 6 days post inoculation, although all had been determined to have the condition earlier in the study.[65]

Vitamin D deficiency (and severe D deficiency such as in rickets) has long been correlated with increased respiratory tract infections,[66] [67] including in this 15-year observational study.[68] In the Martineau-Joliffe study, vitamin D blood levels had statistically significant inverse correlation with mortality from respiratory tract diseases. Darker skin color[69] and advanced age[70] have both been shown to inhibit vitamin D production in the skin. Obesity is inversely correlated with vitamin D levels, because too little of body stores of vitamin D is available outside adipose tissue.[71]

1, 25 (OH)2 cholecalciferol is the active form of vitamin D. Eggs, fish and meat are dietary sources, and high fructose corn syrup is an anti-source in the sense of interfering with active vitamin D. Sunlight is the optimal and universally available source of Vitamin D. This is likely a key and underappreciated aspect of why respiratory viruses have such strong seasonality, and are problematic for humans primarily in the winter and early spring, after the year's fewest hours and lowest angle of sunlight at the winter solstice in each hemisphere respectively. This event corresponds with the time of least endogenous vitamin D production. Humans spend an average of 7 to 8% of our time outdoors.[72] However, for those living north of the 35th parallel in the northern hemisphere, or south of the 35th parallel in the southern hemisphere, our winters expose us to only low angled, indirect rays of sunlight, and residents of those regions are generally not able to acquire enough sunlight to rely on sun exposure alone for adequate production of vitamin D. That is, to have enough vitamin D in those regions of the earth in their respective winters, vitamin D must be supplemented or obtained through diet. Sunlight exposure is further limited by staying inside during harsh weather, and dressing to minimize exposed skin while venturing outdoors. Further since mid-2020, mask-wearing is popular, which further reduces the little available skin to sun exposure and vitamin D availability. This may contribute to the finding that masked populations have been found to have higher rates of COVID-19 than unmasked populations.[73] Vitamin D vs COVID-19 is explored below, now that much research has been produced during 2020 and is available on this topic.

Sanatoriums were the treatment of choice in pandemic tuberculosis treatment. Regular sunlight exposure was a daily component of the treatment there. Vitamin D was gradually reasoned and understood to be essential to conquering the pathogenesis of tuberculosis in these settings. What is now better understood about this effect is as follows: The presence of the Mycobacterium tuberculosis upregulates a key enzyme, CYP27B1 and the vitamin D receptors in macrophages. This has been found to lead to downstream production of the peptide cathelicidin, which is anti-microbial toward the Tuberculosis bacterium,[74] as well as Influenza A,[75] and other bacteria and viruses.[76] However, the association was not observed to hold for Hepatitis B or C, even though all of those patients had lower vitamin D levels than controls.[77] Cathelicidin is able to kill pathogenic viruses and bacteria directly, and it is able to bind to endotoxin, by forming ion channels and increasing membrane permeability. [78] Vitamin D has been established to be key to this process.[79] [80] [81] [82]

Vitamin D and the innate immune system

Vitamin D is active in the innate immune system,[83] Vitamin D interacts with the immune system as it connects with receptors on white blood cells. If the location and function of adaptive immunity can be considered primarily systemic, the location and function of the innate immune system is local everywhere throughout the body. The innate immune system is the first to encounter infection. 1,25 (OH) vitamin D hydroxylase has been found in dendritic cells and macrophages, which are present at the site of first inflammation.[84] In its active form, 1,25 di-hydroxy-vitamin D3, or calcitriol, has receptors in every tissue in the body where it was searched.

In the innate immune system, vitamin D is essential to the maturing of macrophages. Vitamin D was found to cause precursor cells, promyelocytes to differentiate into monocytes.[85] [86] These are precursor cells to macrophages. Activated macrophages influenced by vitamin D produce hydrogen peroxide, which is an important pro-oxidant molecular weapon against pathogenic microbes, including viruses.[87]

Vitamin D receptors have been found throughout the innate immune system in these cellular components: monocytes and macrophages, dendritic cells,[88] as well as in the adaptive immune system, in T cells and B cells.[89] The cells in the innate immune system, epithelial cells in the respiratory tract, as well monocytes, macrophages and dendritic cells were also found to have the enzyme CYP27B1, which is required to convert inactive vitamin D to the active form, 1,25-OH-vitamin D.[90] [91] Vitamin D stimulates a variety of anti-microbial peptides that appear in natural killer cells and neutrophils in respiratory tract epithelial cells, where they have a protective role in lung tissues against the ravages of infection and inflammation.

Inflammatory cytokines are a double-edged sword for the severely ill. While acting as overwhelming forces against pathogenic invasion, the results of cytokine storm can be so overwhelming for the frail patient that they become the immediate cause of death. In these situations also, vitamin D plays a necessary role in prevention of excessive inflammatory cytokines.

Adaptive immunity vs COVID-19

The vaccine manufacturers have focused, as they must in every vaccine for it to address advertised claims, on recognizable proteins produced by a pathogen. In the case of COVID-19, as with other coronaviruses, that protein is a spike protein. Immunologic memory following either naturally acquired infection or the vaccine arouses immunological memory. Then, after a subsequent exposure to the spike protein, you have the expected secondary response.

A secondary response to a pathogen, acquired either naturally or from a vaccine, is a stronger and faster response than in the first encounter. Often these are so fast and forceful that an individual can clear a virus before even being aware of its presence. This is an asymptomatic defeat of the virus. The goal of vaccination is for the vaccinated individual to experience no disease from the pathogen.

A problem with the use of vaccines against COVID-19, is that they were developed for only months prior to use with the public. Professor of viral immunology Byram Bridle discusses how corners were cut, the Phase three clinical trials were skipped, which forced the public on which the vaccines were used to become the phase three clinical trial subjects, of course, unbeknownst to them: "Those being vaccinated now are, whether they realize it or not, part of the phase three experiment.[92]

Adaptive immunity and Vitamin D

Vitamin D receptors have been found in abundance in activated lymphocytes.[93][94] Whereas multiple lymphocytes contain vitamin D receptors, CD-8 lymphocytes, also known as cytotoxic T-cells, were found to have the highest concentration, and vitamin D was found to increase the number of those receptors.[95] However, vitamin D also regulates helper T cells, notably TH1, TH2 and TH17, as well as the regulatory T cells that play an essential role in the prevention of auto-immune disease, as discussed previously. Where vitamin D is deficient, T-lymphocytes are shown to be pathogenic.[96]

TH1 helper T cells tend to be more pro-inflammatory; their cytokines include interleukin (IL)-2, interferon gamma and tumor necrosis factor (TNF)-alpha, and vitamin D tends to suppress TH1, switching adaptive immune response to TH2.[97] For example, the vitamin D receptor (VDR) inhibits the T-cell cytokine IL-2.[98] In contrast, vitamin D tends to enhance TH2 helper T-cell proliferation and cytokine production. TH2 T-cells are more anti-inflammatory and those cells excrete such cytokines as the interleukins IL-3, IL4, IL-5 and IL-10.[99][100]

Vitamin D3 has shown association with priming naïve human T cells, specifically CD4 and CD8 T lymphocytes, to enhance their migration to sites of infection.[101] The expression and activity of vitamin D receptors are important for every stage examined in the life of a T lymphocyte, including development, differentiation and expression of effector functions.[102]

Vitamin D vs viral infections

In the presence of pathogenic respiratory viruses, normal lung epithelial cells convert 25-hydroxy vitamin D (which is the inactive or storage form of vitamin D) to the active form, namely 1,25-

hydroxyvitamin D3, which is the active form.[103] Cathelicidins are stimulated by vitamin D, as discussed above, and are essential to defense against viruses. Vitamin D also stimulates the powerful Type I Interferons (IFNs) which in turn stimulate expression of over 100 IFN stimulated genes, which show a variety of antiviral activities.[104] [105] Vitamin D also showed evidence of inhibiting viral replication.[106]

COVID-19 has been compared to respiratory syncytial virus (RSV) in that both have shown life-threatening amounts of inflammatory chemokines in the airways. In both diseases, this process has been a part of its pathogenesis, severity of the infection and mortality.[107] Modest improvement in each is obtainable with prescribed corticosteroids,[108] but vitamin D gave more consistent response in RSV treatment.[109] Even the intractable human immunodeficiency virus (HIV-1) has shown susceptibility to Vitamin D treatment.[110] [111]

Significantly improved outcomes of respiratory infections have been seen with vitamin D supplementation and / or higher serum levels, in terms of shorter hospitalization, lower cost of care and lower mortality.[112] [113] In a study of 18,883 individuals, there was an increased prevalence of upper respiratory tract infection in those having less than 30 ng/ml serum levels of 25-hydroxy vitamin D compared to those having 30 ng/ml and above. This association was even stronger than season, body mass index, history of asthma or smoking or chronic obstructive pulmonary disease (COPD).[114] Pneumonia patients with < 12 ng/ml 25-hydroxy vitamin D levels had higher mortality at 30 days.[115] Children also showed correlation between low vitamin D levels and pneumonia and acute lower respiratory infection.[116] [117] Likewise, vitamin D deficiency in children was associated with more likelihood of hospitalization, severity of disease and longer hospitalization for respiratory infections.[118]

Vitamin D vs COVID

COVID-19 is widely considered to be a serious disease, with a generally agreed infection fatality rate (IFR) of 0.23%,[119] which is similar to annual influenza IFR. The IFR has recently, as of this writing, been determined to be lower, 0.15%[120] as populations approach herd immunity. This was measured during a year in which treatments that had been well-studied against COVID-19 were rarely used in western hospitals. Because there are a number of well-researched, and widely used therapeutics against COVID-19, and that many of these have been used in the home setting, rather than reported as "cases," it is likely that the true IFR is lower than 0.23%.

Early on in the COVID-19 pandemic, it became clear that the time-honored and well-understood immune-regulatory and anti-viral effect of Vitamin D was clearly applicable as a preventive agent, and many independent clinicians around the world recommended it to our patients, with early support in the medical literature.[121]

However, not all of vitamin D's actions against SARS-CoV-2 has directly involved what is commonly considered the immune system. SARS-CoV-2 enters cells on the ACE-2 receptor. ACE-2 is essential in the renin-angiotensin-aldosterone system (RAAS), typically considered primarily involved in homeostasis of sodium, water and blood pressure. But RAAS is also present in the cells of the lungs' alveoli, and is closely correlated with lung imjury.[122] ACE was found to be significantly elevated in COVID-19 diagnosed patients.[123] Vitamin D thwarts this SARS-CoV-2 invasive mechanism by inhibiting renin production in the kidneys.

COVID-19 shows a similar demographic profile of mortality as the vitamin D-deficient cohorts, affecting those of advanced age, darker skin color, and higher BMI than other populations, in this study of 17,278,392 patients, examining over 10,000 deaths.[124] A CDC study found 78% of people who were hospitalized for COVID were overweight or obese.[125] Geographic distribution away from the equator was positively correlated with COVID-19 mortality rates. In fact, all countries within 35 degrees latitude away from the equator have had low mortality from COVID-19.[126] In twenty European countries, a significant inverse relationship was found between serum vitamin D levels and COVID-19 mortality. Aging populations, which have had the most severe COVID-19 experiences, were found to have the lowest mean serum levels of vitamin D.[127]

People with positive PCR results for COVID-19 had statistically significant low vitamin D serum levels compared to those with negative PCR test results.[128] [129] [130] [131] However, this may have been due to an expected drop in vitamin D after infection. However, in a study of 14,000 patients in Israel, who had previously measured vitamin D levels, it was found that even prior, rather than current, high levels of vitamin D were associated with almost no COVID-19 hospitalization, especially in the over 60 age group.[132] It was remarkable that vitamin D levels over 75 nmol/l were associated with exceptionally little COVID-19 in seniors. Regardless of age, gender and comorbidities, in a university hospital study in Germany of 185 patients, who were diagnosed with and treated for COVID-19, there was 80% less risk of ventilator need and 90% lower mortality among those with adequate vitamin D levels.[133] In a much larger study of over 190,000 people in the US, vitamin D levels measured in the serum were strongly inversely related to SARS-CoV-2 positive PCR test results, regardless of age, race, gender and geographic area of residence. Here is their graph of results:[134]

© Kaufman, Niles, et al. Endnote 134.

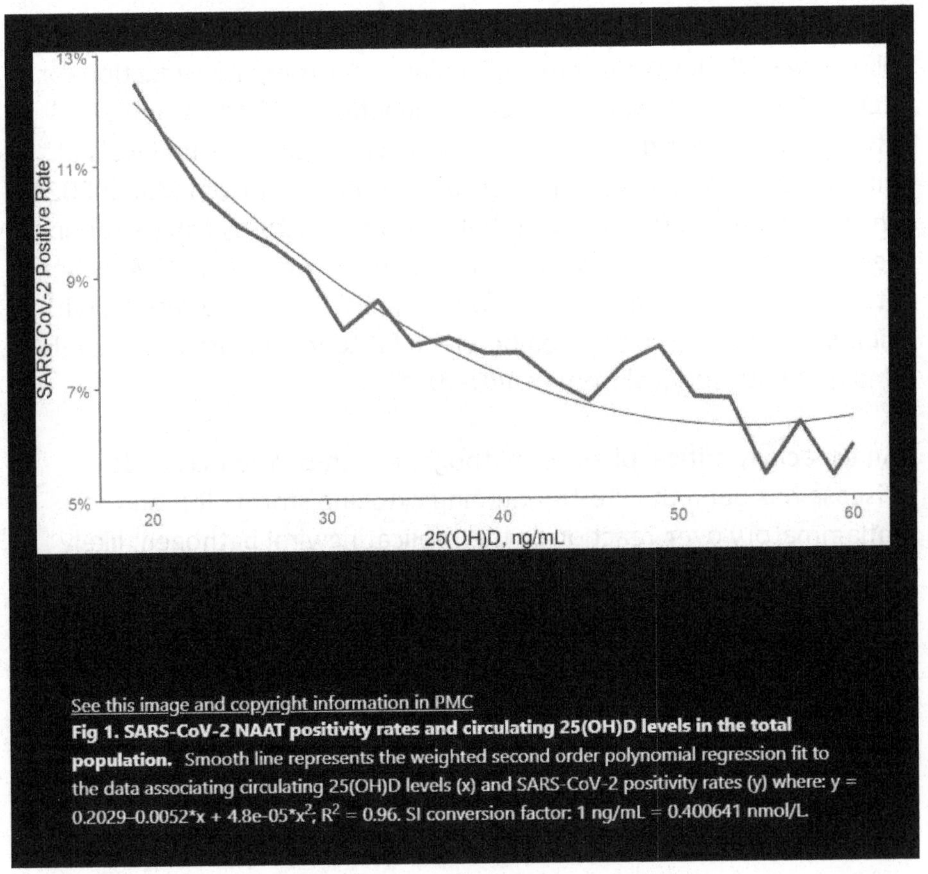

See this image and copyright information in PMC

Fig 1. SARS-CoV-2 NAAT positivity rates and circulating 25(OH)D levels in the total population. Smooth line represents the weighted second order polynomial regression fit to the data associating circulating 25(OH)D levels (x) and SARS-CoV-2 positivity rates (y) where: $y = 0.2029 - 0.0052 * x + 4.8e\text{-}05 * x^2$; $R^2 = 0.96$. SI conversion factor: 1 ng/mL = 0.400641 nmol/L.

A study of people testing positive for COVID-19 in India found that those with higher vitamin D levels were significantly more likely to be asymptomatic than those with lower levels. In that study, of hospitalized COVID-19 patients, those with normal vitamin D levels had 15% of the mortality rate of those with low vitamin D levels.[135]

Mortality of hospitalized COVID-19 patients has been found to be significantly higher among those with lower serum vitamin D levels.[136] [137] [138] Conversely, vitamin D was positively correlated with survival of hospitalized COVID-19 patients, in alignment with prior and worldwide results. Another study of 551 COVID-19 patients showed strong correlation between low vitamin D levels and mortality, even more strongly associated than BMI and mortality.[139] Over 1500 patients across five UK hospitals showed similar and strong risk reduction for COVID-19 mortality with supplemented vitamin D3.[140] A similar US study also showed decreased mortality with higher serum levels of vitamin D.[141] An analysis of 19 European countries from March 2021 through January 2021 showed that lower mean 25-hydroxy vitamin D serum levels correlated with higher COVID-19 mortality.[142] Another study of 18 European countries found similar COVID-19 results, with a significant inverse correlation between latitude and vitamin D levels, and also with survival from COVID-19.[143]

An especially critical phase of pathogenesis in severe COVID-19 disease has been the life-threatening cytokine storm. It is an inflammatory over-reaction to the replicating viral pathogen, likely more pronounced due to its late onset, discussed above. Vitamin D may have a crucial role in prevention of excessive inflammatory cytokines.[144] [145] [146] [147]

Is it possible that COVID-19 is another name for a deficiency of vitamin D?[148] Acute Respiratory Distress Syndrome (ARDS) is the most iconic characteristic of SARS (Severe Acute Respiratory Syndrome). Vitamin D deficiency was found to be common in people who develop ARDS.[149] [150] Severe acute hypoxemia was correlated with low vitamin D levels in this retrospective study of 348 hospitalized patients in Italy.[151]

How much vitamin D is optimal to take?

Endemic vitamin D deficiency is widespread in many countries,[152] especially among seniors in nursing homes,[153] dating from before the COVID-19 phenomenon. Non-equatorial populations have less vitamin D available in the winter.[154] Winter presents a trifecta of vitamin D challenges: First, there are fewer hours of sunlight. Second the sun is lower in the sky, its rays not so direct on the skin as during summer. Third, we bundle up against cold weather, leaving minimal skin exposed while outdoors. All of these reduce opportunity to begin vitamin D production in the skin. Use of facemasks further reduces skin available for vitamin D production.

Therefore, during a time of low availability of sunlight for endogenous vitamin D production, it is likely prudent to supplement this nutrient. Single bolus dosing of vitamin D3 did not help hospitalized patients with severe COVID-19.[155] However, in a double-blind trial, when patients who were hospitalized with acute COVID-19 received 3 or more doses of calcifediol (25-OH vitamin D, which is a pre-cursor to the active form 1,25-OH vitamin D3), the need for intensive care treatment was significantly reduced to only one of 50 patients, and none in the treatment group died, whereas half of the control patients were admitted to intensive care.[156] Vitamin D supplementation reduced inflammatory markers in COVID-19 patients.[157]

Vitamin D is a fat soluble vitamin, and therefore not so quickly metabolized and excreted from the body as are water soluble vitamins, such as the B family and C vitamins. Still, regular supplementation seems to be more effective than seldom boluses. In one study, an enormous initial dose of 200,000 IU, followed by 100,000 IU once per month, resulted in no decrease of severity or incidence of respiratory infections than the control group.[158] In contrast, to such seldom dosing, daily dosing of vitamin D was associated with better outcomes against Influenza A[159] and other respiratory infections, even as low as 400 IU/day to 2000 IU/day, as in this meta-analysis.[160] 800 IU Vitamin D3 has been associated with decreased incidence of bone fracture.[161] Such doses are generally considered to be unacceptably low doses among naturopathic physicians, and too low generally to be effective against viral infections such as COVID-19.

Vitamin D has a long history of beneficial effect against cancer. In the author's cancer clinic, 14 years of daily direct contact with and clinical treatment of cancer patients has relied on daily dosing of 8,000 to 10,000 units of vitamin D3, and has been correlated, among use of many other nutrients, with extraordinary success in both remission from cancer and lack of cancer recurrence.[162] No signs of intolerance of vitamin D3, nor of hyper-vitaminosis of vitamin D or hypercalcemia (that wasn't already associated with osseous metastases or with hyperparathyroidism) has been seen in the clinic over those 14 years. Therefore, the author and colleagues have generally considered this to be a safe and effective dose for themselves as well, and we have often taken that daily dose also, though generally not so consistently as our cancer patients.

Even at supplementation of 20,000 IU per day of vitamin D3, it was found that Canadian adults had no evidence of vitamin D toxicity.[163] Toxicity that was associated with vitamin D supplementation was found to be extremely rare, and in each case to be accompanied by calcium supplementation.[164] [165]

Supplementation of vitamin D was significantly associated with lower rates of COVID-19 cases in univariate analysis,[166] but not multivariate analysis.[167] The sample size was 349,598 participants with known baseline vitamin D levels, compiled from years earlier.

How urgent is it for people all over the world to have access to sufficient vitamin D?

Much of the western hemisphere, and people in countries throughout the world have been traumatized by the COVID-19 phenomenon, with fear of death rivalling and likely surpassing the pathogenicity of the associated SARS-CoV-2 virus. Populations across the world have submitted to the extraordinary measures imposed by their governments to attempt to thwart the feared pandemic. These efforts have largely failed for reasons given in Part 2 of this book.

Vitamin D, on the other hand, might be called a Godsend by some, and should be recognized by now as a necessary nutrient for immune function, and a specifically useful and decisive one in defeating COVID-19, as we see study after study above, from small to enormous, showing -- not just significantly – but drastically improved outcomes for those who supplement vitamin D before and during their experience with COVID-19. To achieve adequate vitamin D levels, particularly during fall, winter and spring, when seasonal respiratory viruses are most active, supplementation is highly recommended for everyone. Vitamin D supplementation should be kept in adequate supply in every household, especially as it moves into winter, and to be sure there is enough for daily use for every household member, as an easy preventive measure, with no known drawback to daily use. The urgency of such widespread vitamin D availability and storage, particularly for the COVID era, cannot be overemphasized, and epidemiologist Hermann Brenner makes a strong case for it here.[168]

It would be quite difficult for a person with adequate serum vitamin D levels to die of COVID-19. How difficult is it?

Mayo Clinic found "Among patients admitted with laboratory-confirmed COVID-19, 25 (OH) D levels were inversely associated with in-hospital mortality and the need for invasive mechanical ventilation."[169] In this study of 120 already severe cases of COVID-19 in Algeria, it was also found that those with the lowest vitamin D levels were the most likely to die with a COVID-19 diagnosis.[170] Here is the graph of that correlation.

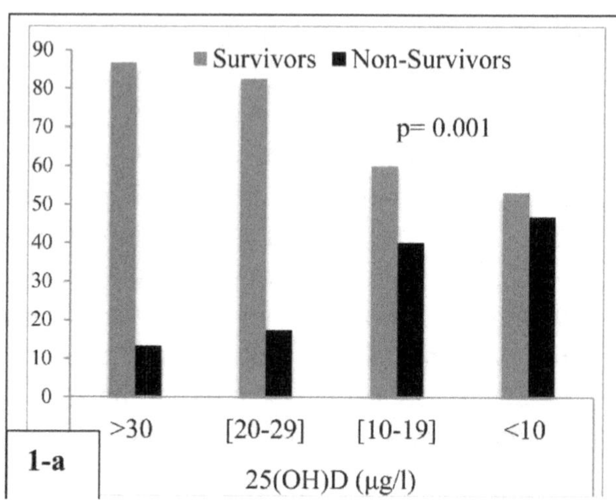

Graph © S Bennouar, A Cherif, et al.

At this writing, the world population is 7,853,464,319 and the number of deaths attributed to COVID-19 is 2,716,882. Therefore, 0.000345947, which is about 0.0346% of the world's citizens have been alleged to die from COVID-19. Considering that even among those with diagnosis of severe COVID-19 illness, represented in the above graph, only 10% of those with the modest vitamin D level of > 30 ng/ml died with a COVID-19 diagnosis, and the other 90% survived, then it is exceedingly difficult to die of COVID-19 with adequate vitamin D levels.

Studies from all over the world show significantly and overwhelmingly lower rates of death in COVID-19 patients with adequate vitamin D levels. Here is a visual representation of those linked, mostly peer-reviewed, studies from the compendium site https://c19vitamind.com. All of the studies shown in the graph below are of diagnosed and/or hospitalized patients with a diagnosis of COVID-19.

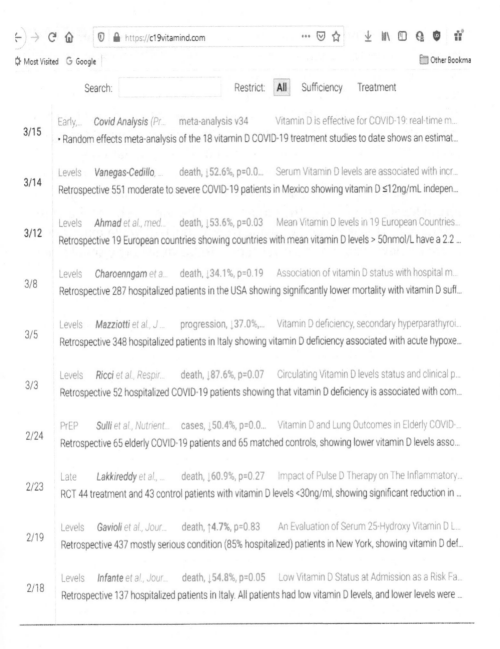

https://c19vitamind.com

Most Visited Google Other Bookma

Search: Restrict: **All** Sufficiency Treatment

Date	Type	Study	Result	Title / Summary
3/15	Early,...	*Covid Analysis* (Pr...	meta-analysis v34	Vitamin D is effective for COVID-19: real-time m... • Random effects meta-analysis of the 18 vitamin D COVID-19 treatment studies to date shows an estimat...
3/14	Levels	*Vanegas-Cedillo*, ...	death, ↓52.6%, p=0.0...	Serum Vitamin D levels are associated with incr... Retrospective 551 moderate to severe COVID-19 patients in Mexico showing vitamin D ≤12ng/mL indepen...
3/12	Levels	*Ahmad* et al., med...	death, ↓53.6%, p=0.03	Mean Vitamin D levels in 19 European Countries... Retrospective 19 European countries showing countries with mean vitamin D levels > 50nmol/L have a 2.2 ...
3/8	Levels	*Charoenngam* et a...	death, ↓34.1%, p=0.19	Association of vitamin D status with hospital m... Retrospective 287 hospitalized patients in the USA showing significantly lower mortality with vitamin D suff...
3/5	Levels	*Mazziotti* et al., J ...	progression, ↓37.0%,...	Vitamin D deficiency, secondary hyperparathyroi... Retrospective 348 hospitalized patients in Italy showing vitamin D deficiency associated with acute hypoxe...
3/3	Levels	*Ricci* et al., Respir...	death, ↓87.6%, p=0.07	Circulating Vitamin D levels status and clinical p... Retrospective 52 hospitalized COVID-19 patients showing that vitamin D deficiency is associated with com...
2/24	PrEP	*Sulli* et al., Nutrient...	cases, ↓50.4%, p=0.0...	Vitamin D and Lung Outcomes in Elderly COVID-... Retrospective 65 elderly COVID-19 patients and 65 matched controls, showing lower vitamin D levels asso...
2/23	Late	*Lakkireddy* et al., ...	death, ↓60.9%, p=0.27	Impact of Pulse D Therapy on The Inflammatory... RCT 44 treatment and 43 control patients with vitamin D levels <30ng/ml, showing significant reduction in ...
2/19	Levels	*Gavioli* et al., Jour...	death, ↑4.7%, p=0.83	An Evaluation of Serum 25-Hydroxy Vitamin D L... Retrospective 437 mostly serious condition (85% hospitalized) patients in New York, showing vitamin D def...
2/18	Levels	*Infante* et al., Jour...	death, ↓54.8%, p=0.05	Low Vitamin D Status at Admission as a Risk Fa... Retrospective 137 hospitalized patients in Italy. All patients had low vitamin D levels, and lower levels were ...

A diagnosis of COVID-19, currently defined by governments and media as a "case," whether sick or well, is already shown in the studies above to be rare with adequate vitamin D levels.[171] [172] [173] [174] Symptomatic expression of COVID-19 is still less likely with adequate Vitamin D levels.[175] Hospitalization and mortality with COVID-19 patients has been found to be significantly lower among those with adequate serum vitamin D levels.[176] [177] [178] Each of these studies examined different serum levels of vitamin D among people in different parts of the world, with varying access to sunlight, with or without dosing of vitamin D, and with varying intervals of dosing. The data taken together, however, make a strong case for the difficulty of actually dying of COVID-19 while maintaining adequate vitamin D levels. The serum levels observed in the studies cited herein rarely reached into >70 ng/ml. The likelihood of dying from COVID-19 while maintaining vitamin D levels above this level seems to be vanishingly small if not impossible.

Vitamin C vs COVID

Vitamin C is "the ultimate virucide"

Vitamin C is a vitamin, at least for humans, because it is a vital nutrient, required to be supplied from the diet. Humans and other primates are in the minority among animal species, in that we do not make vitamin C in the body, due to a mutation occurring in our early ancestors. In physically, microbially or psychologically stressful situations, our bodies rapidly deplete vitamin C stores, unfortunately when we need them the most. People deficient in vitamin C are especially susceptible to respiratory conditions including pneumonia,[179] [180] which is alleviated by supplementation of vitamin C.[181]

Vitamin C has been so successful against pneumonia that three different randomized clinical trials found a greater than 80% lower incidence of pneumonia for the oral vitamin C group.[182] [183] [184]

Vitamin C should be no surprise as an addition to the list of nutrients that are useful against COVID-19. Dr. Fred Klenner wrote in 1948 about use of intravenous and intramuscular use of vitamin C against viral pneumonia: "In almost every case the patient felt better within an hour after the first injection and noted a very definite change after two hours." [185] And "three to seven injections gave complete clinical and x-ray response in all of our [42] cases."

Dr. Thomas Levy writes: "As the ultimate virucide, vitamin C has been documented to inactivate or destroy every virus against which it was tested in vitro. Similarly, vitamin C has consistently resolved nearly all acute viral infections in patients treated with sufficient doses." He discusses these clinical findings extensively here [186] and here. [187] Animal studies show that vitamin C reduces both incidence and severity of viral and bacterial infections.[188]

Vitamin C has numerous well-studied and documented mechanisms against viruses. Perhaps the most important of these is the production of Type I interferons.[189] This in turn upregulates natural killer cells and cytotoxic T-lymphocytes for anti-viral activity.[190] However, it has been shown to simply inactivate both RNA and DNA viruses.[191] It also detoxifies viral products that are associated with inflammation and pain. High dose vitamin C and oral doses over 3 grams are established to both prevent and treat a variety of viral infections.[192] [193]

Vitamin C vs COVID 19

There is a tendency for lower serum vitamin C levels in many of the same demographic groups that have the highest incidence of COVID-19: male, African American, older, patients with co-morbidities, particularly diabetes, COPD and hypertension.[194] [195] This raises the question of to what extent COVID-19 may be a disease of vitamin C deficiency, or a manifestation of an early stage of the lethal disease known as scurvy.

Vitamin C was observed to be deficient in COVID-19 patients, on average only 22% of the serum levels of healthy controls (11.4 µmol/L vs 52 µmol/L). High dose IV vitamin C raised the COVID-19 group to normal range of 76 µmol/L).[196] The authors went so far to conclude that "vitamin C supplementation is necessary for patients with coronavirus disease." Plasma levels of vitamin C are considered deficient if less than 11.4 µmol /L, and more than 7% of US citizens,

>20 million people in the USA are below this level.[197] People of low income and smokers are more likely to be deficient.[198]

At the Ruijing Hospital in Shanghai, 50 COVID-19 patients were treated with vitamin C. Their hospital stays were 5 days shorter than those COVID-19 patients not treated with Vitamin C. There were no deaths in the Vitamin C group, and no significant side effects were noted either. All patients in that group were discharged. In the other group of COVID-19 patients, those who did not receive vitamin C, there were 3 deaths.[199]

Dr. Zhiyong Peng conducted the first clinical trial of high-dose intravenous vitamin C with COVID-19 patients at Wuhan University in Wuhan, China. His findings were that this treatment of COVID-19 patients reduced their inflammation significantly, and that it reduced their stays in ICU and hospitals.[200] [201]

A randomized controlled trial in Wuhan, China, with critically ill COVID-19 patients on ventilators were treated with a placebo or vitamin C, 24 g/day for 7 days. Mortality at 28 days was 18% in the treatment group vs 50% in the control group.[202] When vitamin C doses were smaller the improvement in mortality was less successful. In a UK study, one gram of intravenous vitamin C given every 12 hours with anticoagulants only improved mortality from 41% of ICU COVID-19 patients to 29% mortality.[203] [204] With COVID-19 patients in ICUs in Texas and Virginia, doses of intravenous vitamin C at 1.5 g every 6 hours lowered mortality to 5%, which was the lowest of any hospital in their respective counties.[205]

Vitamin C was found to be associated with duration of symptoms in COVID-19 patients from 9 days in the control arm to 6 days in the treatment arm, which was a 33% reduction in symptom duration.[206] A study of hospitalized patients in Pakistan showed 26% faster recovery and 36% lower mortality from COVID-19 than controls.[207] In another study without a control group, COVID-19 pneumonia patients who were in severe or critical condition were given high dose IV vitamin C.

Improvements were seen in arterial oxygen, organ function and levels of lymphocytes generally and CD4+ T cell counts in particular. Arterial oxygen normalized by the 3rd day in severe patients and by day 7 in critical patients.[208]

Mechanisms of Vitamin C vs COVID-19

Fulminant COVID-19 disease is characterized by a strongly destabilized immune / inflammatory imbalance. This is characterized by such pro-inflammatory cytokines as interleukin 6 (IL-6) in the body. Cytokine storm is often observed as well, characterized by proliferation of neutrophils in the lungs, which burst capillaries in the alveoli. In contrast, vitamin C reduces these pro-inflammatory cytokines, and down-regulates the activation and proliferation of neutrophils and neutrophil extracellular traps.[209]

SARS-CoV-2 downregulates Type-1 interferons (INF-1),[210] which is one of our strongest anti-viral defenses. Vitamin C has the opposite effect; it upregulates INF-1.[211]

SARS-CoV-2 enters human cells via the ACE-2 receptor, and severe COVID-19 disease is correlated with upregulated ACE-2, as in hypertension and cardiovascular disease. In fact, during a year of intense confusion of what patient pathology may be attributed to what cause of death, it has been observed that deaths of heart disease have been among the most likely to be mistakenly attributed to COVID-19 deaths. [212] The SARS-CoV-2 spike glycoprotein binds to ACE2.[213] However, vitamin C was found to decisively reverse ACE2 increase by means of the interleukin IL-7.[214]

There is some evidence for Vitamin C having the following mechanisms against COVID-19 pathology: interferon production, improvement of the lung epithelial barrier, reduction of NF-kB signaling, and reduction of neutrophil extracellular trap formation.[215]

Oral dosing of vitamin C

As shown above, the strongest and fastest effects of vitamin C against COVID-19 were observed with high dose intravenous vitamin C. These may safely – subject to the following metabolic limitations - go up to about 25 g, 35 g or somewhat higher per dose, provided osmolarity limits are considered, and depending on individual tolerance, but beyond that is considered to be too hyperosmolar in most administered mixtures, at least by this author, who has used vitamin C intravenously tens of thousands of times with patients since 2006.[216] Before high doses of vitamin C are administered, it is necessary to check the patient for normal glucose-6 phosphate dehydrogenase (G6PD) and a history of thalassemia. Even these are not absolute deterrents to high dose vitamin C if properly administered with complementary nutrients as determined by the naturopathic physician or other knowledgeable healthcare provider.

For prophylactic dosing at well tolerated limits, two to 8 grams per day are sometimes taken orally in divided doses, if done in consultation with a naturopathic physician, or other knowledgeable healthcare provider. It must be kept in mind that as of this writing, there is inadequate to non-existent nutrition education in the conventional medical curriculum, and therefore, it is important for patients to learn if their healthcare provider has had multiple courses in nutrition, as advanced and applied biochemistry, throughout medical school.

Despite early suspicions that high doses of vitamin C could cause kidney stones, those hypotheses have since been disproven, and that the earlier studies had faulty designs.[217] [218] Because of such misconceptions and fears, the lives lost from inadequate dosing of vitamin C to pneumonia and COVID-19 patients must be considered seriously in future research and clinical practice.

Clinicians treating severely ill COVID-19 patients found clinical effects on giving 3 grams of vitamin C every 6 hours, together with steroids, vitamin B1 and anti-coagulants.[219]

It took hundreds of years for naval captains throughout the North Atlantic to fully recognize the essential addition to sailors' diet of citrus and other high vitamin C foods, in order to prevent their deaths from the dreaded scurvy on long ocean voyages. Vitamin C was only recognized much later as the key necessary ingredient in such foods, and later still came the knowledge that vitamin C is required by the body to form collagen, the most common protein in our tissues. Without adequate replacement of that protein as our cells turn over, tissue becomes fragile, weak and easily breached. This is why sailors' scurvy resulted in bleeding gums before other symptoms were noted.

Contemporary populations once again forget humanity's everlasting dependence on external sources of vitamin C, a substance that we cannot make in our bodies, but must obtain through diet. As the natural whole vegetables and fruits and organ meats that are abundant in vitamin C take a small role in the 20th and 21st century diet, people once again suffer the consequences of that loss. Perhaps COVID-19 is only the latest reminder of the devastation suffered by people who are critically deficient in this vital nutrient.

Zinc vs COVID

Although zinc is the second most abundant metal in humans, zinc deficiency is very common, and in developing countries it is the 5th leading cause of death for loss of life years. Approximately 2 billion people worldwide are affected by zinc deficiency.[220] Red meat and oysters, are among the most luxury foods on the planet and are highest in zinc. Legumes and other phytates, which are more ubiquitous in human diet throughout the world, bind zinc, making it less available. In industrial countries, mainly the elderly are zinc deficient.[221] Supplementation of 45 mg zinc per day, over 12 months was correlated with a significant reduction in incidence of infections generally, and was very well tolerated in a senior population.[222]

The amount of zinc in a human cell is limited, possibly to < 1000 atoms per cell, although that number is controversial, partly because zinc plays a role in normal cell death.[223] [224] A survival mechanism of a normal cell is therefore to limit the zinc that can enter by means of metallothionein binding, balanced against zinc transporter activity. Zinc importers (primarily ZIP proteins) and zinc exporters (primarily ZnT proteins) have rival activity, called "muffling," which keeps a cytotoxic amount of metal out of the cell, but a nourishing amount in. More than 30 known proteins perform this function of zinc homeostasis, which harmoniously ensure that zinc levels do not rise above toxic thresholds, nor fail to rise to a minimal adequacy.[225] [226] Even with this system of checks and balances, zinc is sequestered in vesicles known as zincosomes (50%) and 30-40% is in the cytoplasm.[227]

A nourishing or necessary amount of zinc is that which supports and regulates enzyme structure, catalysis and transcription.[228]

Zinc is required in both the innate and adaptive immune systems. Transcription factors that carry zinc impact both the innate and adaptive immune systems, and impact cell development.229 Zinc is necessary for functions of mast cells,[230] as well as monocytes[231] and macrophages.[232] [233] Zinc is important to the function of dendritic cells.[234] Zinc is key to the functions of neutrophils, such as phagocytosis and degranulation, as well as cytokine production, secretion and function, as well as chemotaxis.[235] Natural killer cell function and recognition of major histocompatibility complex class 1 (MHC-1) depends on adequate zinc.[236] [237]

Zinc's role in adaptive immune function is appreciated by observing changes in zinc deficient individuals. Here we see lymphopenia[238] and reduced proportion of helper T cells to cytotoxic T cells.[239] One reason for these deficiencies is that zinc is necessary for the maturation and differentiation of T and B cells. Zinc supplementation has been shown to restore activity of the thymus.[240] B cells' development and function are impacted by the presence of zinc.[241] [242]

Thus, here is yet another nutrient, with immune function far broader than any vaccine ever developed, necessarily, because as we should all know, there is much more to immunity than just antibodies. As we see, "Instead of assigning all the necessary [immune] functions to one single cell type, the immune response is optimized by the cooperation of various cell types, supported by soluble mediators with distinct functions, roughly separated into innate, fast responding cells and highly specific adaptive immune cells," and "zinc is crucial for the appropriate development and function of the whole immune system, including innate as well as adaptive immunity . . . "[243]

Zinc has many functions in the cell, including RNA transcription and DNA synthesis. Zinc not only has antiviral effect, but it is considered to be physiologically necessary for an effective antiviral response.[244] The beauty of zinc is that it works in favor of the host for these functions, but works against those same functions with respect to pathogenic viruses, basically chopping RNA in the "wrong places" for viral replication, and bringing viral replication to a standstill. This is certainly a wonderful way to defeat SARS-CoV-2 and other pathogens. Specifically, in this case, zinc inhibits replication of RNA-type viruses. SARS-CoV-2 is such a virus. The mechanism is that zinc blocks the enzyme RNA-dependent RNA polymerase (RdRp).245 This enzyme is required for replication of the virus. Without this enzyme, copying of the viral RNA cannot occur. In vitro, zinc also inhibited SARS-CoV-1 RNA polymerase.[246] SARS-Co-V-1 is thought to share most of its genome with SARS-CoV-2, the infectious agent to which COVID-19 is attributed. It is thought that zinc's impairment of the replication of RNA viruses is due to this mechanism: Zinc interferes with and creates errors in proteolytic effects on viral replicase polyproteins,[247] including in coronaviruses.[248] [249] The effect of zinc on coronavirus replication appears to be by both of the above mechanisms.[250]

One of our first clues that zinc may be helpful in COVID-19, is that 16% of all lower respiratory infections world-wide are attributed to zinc deficiency.[251]

Researchers Inga Wessels, Benjamin Rolles and Lothar Rink of Aachen University Faculty of Medicine in Aachen, Germany illustrate the great variety of zinc functions that are applicable and possibly beneficial to COVID-19 patients.[252]

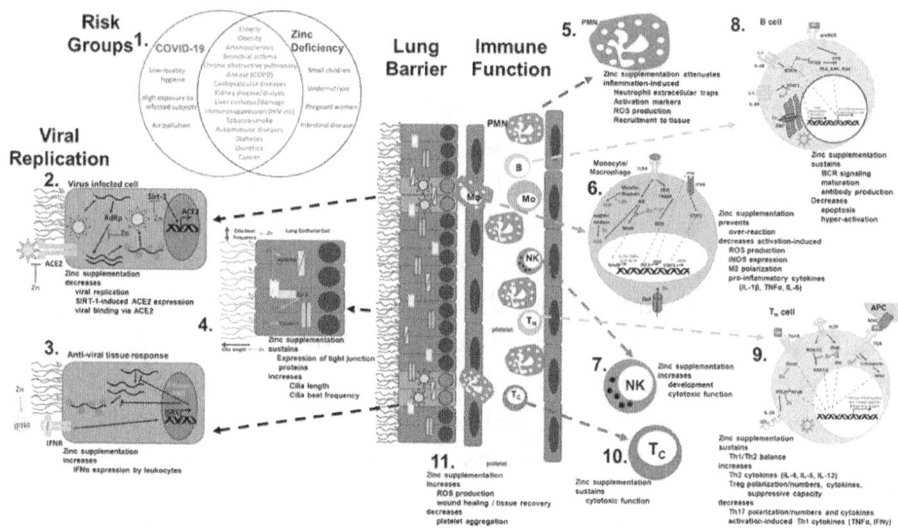

Illustration © Inga Wessels, Benjamin Rolles, Lothar Rink

Besides all of the specific immune effects of zinc discussed above, zinc also contributes to multiple physical barriers against virus entry to the cell. We see in #2 above, zinc inhibits viral binding to the ACE-2 receptor. This is the receptor that SARS-CoV-2 uses to enter cells. It had been thought that ACE-2 was only in different organs, but it has been found in abundance in the epithelia of human lungs and small intestines.[253]

We see that in #4 above that zinc sustains tissue integrity[254] and increases ciliary length, [255] which both act against penetration of viruses beyond epithelial surfaces. Regarding the up- and down-regulation of cells and cell functions, some of which appear contradictory on first observation, Wessels et al explain that zinc is not so much activating or inhibiting of immune function, but that it "normalizes overshooting reactions and balances the ratios of various immune cell types."[256] From the multiple functions shown above of zinc thwarting the SARS-CoV-2 virus and its replication, it would seem that the virus's assault against the body is not merely inhibited, but that it is stopped with adequate zinc.

Zinc deficiency results in a pro-inflammatory phenotype that is similar in several ways to that of severe COVID-19 disease. These include proliferation of pro-inflammatory cytokines, such as IL-6, C-reactive protein and tumor necrosis factor, as well as a reduction in the regulatory T-cells that modulate inflammatory processes. As a result, zinc deficient patients in severe distress suffer from acute respiratory distress syndrome, as well as possibly permanent lung damage and death following systemic inflammation. All of these are coincident with COVID-19 also, as established by numerous studies.[257] [258]

Empirically, we see that zinc deficiency is associated with mortality risk and organ failure in intensive care units generally.[259] [260] For COVID-19 patients, zinc deficiency on admission seemed to these researchers "to provide the most valuable information about disease course and prognosis." [261] In their study, patients with diagnosed COVID-19, zinc serum levels were 26% lower than in healthy controls. Of those who died during the study, 73.5% were below 638.7 µg/L, considered a threshold for zinc deficiency. However, only 40.9% of the survivors were below that level. A retrospective study of 62 hospitalized COVID-19 patients showed average serum zinc levels significantly lower for those requiring intubation versus higher zinc levels in mild and moderate cases.[262]

In another study of 47 COVID-19 patients, those who were zinc deficient were more likely to develop more complications (70.4%) than those within normal range for zinc (30%). Their hospital stays were longer, and they were far more likely to have acute respiratory distress syndrome (ARDS) than those with normal zinc serum levels (18.5% vs 0%).[263]

In another study, COVID-19 patients with significantly lower blood zinc levels had worse clinical outcomes. In this study of 275 patients, average zinc level was 840 µg/L in those with worse outcomes. Those with better clinical outcomes averaged 970 µg/L.[264]

It should also be noted that zinc deficiency is characterized by loss of senses of smell and/or taste. [265] These are also known to be common symptoms of COVID-19 patients.[266] Additional overlapping symptoms between zinc deficiency and COVID-19 are fever, cough, aching limbs and occasionally diarrhea.[267] This is further evidence that deficiency of zinc may be correlated with COVID-19 morbidity. Is this yet another nutrient, besides vitamin D and vitamin C, in which the deficiency is known by another name, that is, COVID-19?

Zinc ionophores

Zinc threshold for antiviral effect may exceed typical physiological concentrations. Whereas zinc levels in human plasma range from 10 to 18 μM,[268] the level of zinc observed in vitro can be in the mM realm.[269] This may be important to understanding the role of zinc ionophores.

In the event of infection with an RNA virus, a useful strategy for medical treatment may be to increase zinc uptake by cells in order to more fully block viral replication. What is needed is a substance that can accompany and transport zinc across the cell membrane and into the cell. Such a substance is an ionophore; it transports the zinc ion. The function is to allow more zinc into a cell than would typically enter. For this purpose, zinc ionophore agents are used in clinical settings together with zinc as a combination strategy against an RNA virus infection.

Zinc and Hydroxychloroquine vs COVID

Hydroxychloroquine (HCQ) is a metabolite of chloroquine (CQ), but each is considered here with regard to its use as an exogenous drug. Both HCQ and its historical predecessor chloroquine CQ are on the World Health Organization's List of Essential Medicines. The latter was discovered in 1934, and it is still used to manage malaria, although resistant strains of malaria make it somewhat less useful these days for that purpose. HCQ has been approved by the US Food and Drug Administration (FDA) for over 65 years. It has been prescribed billions of times throughout the world over the previous decades. The US Centers for Disease Control says that HCQ can be prescribed to adults and children of all ages. It can also be safely taken by pregnant women and nursing mothers.[270] It is among the safest of prescription drugs in the US, which is why it is sold over the counter (not in the US, but) through much of the world.[271]

Both HCQ and CQ are chemically similar to quinine, from the bark of Cinchona trees, which is also a flavoring used in tonic water. Quinine has been appreciated for antiviral activity since at least the 19th century. "The remedy that is most deserving of confidence in the treatment of influenza is quinine. It seems to be really an anti-toxin in this disease."[272] The US National Institute of Health (NIH) under Dr. Anthony Fauci, is in 2020-2021 ideologically opposed to the use of CQ or HCQ for treatments of SARS-CoV-2 infections. However, in 2005, the same NIH had found such strong in vitro results of CQ against SARS that they had this to say on its value: "Our data provide evidence for the possibility of using the well-established drug chloroquine in the clinical management of SARS." They found that it was "likely to have both prophylactic and therapeutic advantages," and found therapeutic plasma concentrations to be achievable, while being well-tolerated.[273] About 30% of common cold infections are coronaviruses; they are not new to humanity. Nor are positive-sense, single-stranded, beta coronaviruses, such as SARS-CoV-2. In 1889, Edwin Wiley Grove marketed Grove's Laxative Bromo Quinine tablets as a common cold remedy. Within 11 years, his company was the largest consumer of quinine in the world.[274]

However, the most useful application of hydroxychloroquine in our time, and in parts of the world worst affected by seasonal virus outbreaks and epidemics may be in the multiple anti-viral mechanisms of HCQ and CQ.[275] [276]

These alkaline drugs are easily taken up into the cells of the body. They have been observed to raise the pH of the cell generally, but also to accumulate inside endosomes, and to alkalinize endosomes and lysosomes in which entering viruses are packaged.[277] Endosomes are abundant in lung tissue, but especially in alveolar cells.[278] Chloroquine is the most thoroughly studied lysosomotropic drug that accomplishes the effect of neutralizing the acidic pH of acidic organelles such as endosomes and lysosomes that transport viruses.[279] Viruses, including coronaviruses, enter cells packaged in endosomes, and require a low pH acidic environment in the endosome in order to function.[280] Once HCQ or CQ are inside cells, these drugs easily enter endosomes, and therefore viruses are stopped from replicating, due to this alkalinizing effect.[281] The specific interference in the replication of SARS-CoV-2 is that HCQ / CQ stops fusion and uncoating.[282] This is considered to be the strongest or one of the strongest effects of HCQ / CQ on SARS-CoV-2 infected patients.[283]

Another mechanism of high pH HCQ / CQ is that the entry of SARS CoV-2 to a cell requires cleavage of the S-protein, in order for the virus to enter a cell, and that this process is pH-dependent.[284] [285] A high pH stops the protease activity required for S protein cleavage at the ACE-2 binding site, which inhibits entry to the cell.[286]

The zinc ionophoric mechanism is such that HCQ and CQ shepherd zinc into the cell, and the use of each of these drugs is correlated with higher concentrations of zinc inside cells.[287] Zinc has multiple anti-viral mechanisms, as shown in the previous chapter. As viruses are contained within lysosomes, the value of HCQ /CQ is that they induce accumulation of intracellular zinc ions preferentially inside lysosomes, and that this is accomplished specifically by transporting zinc into cells, rather than simply enhancing intracellular zinc levels.[288]

Another mechanism of HCQ is that it binds to two domains of the SARS-CoV-2 nucleocapsid (N) protein, one of which is an RNA-binding domain. This in turn disrupts interaction with nucleic acids and the liquid-liquid separation phase (LLPS), which is necessary to continue the viral life cycle.[289]

CQ has shown immunomodulatory effects, as it suppresses IL-6 and TNF-alpha. This is helpful to reduce inflammation associated with a number of viral diseases.

Hydroxychloroquine clinical results

HCQ used together with zinc is showing impressive and consistent results around the world against COVID-19, reversing this disease promptly and completely in individuals treated with this protocol. Early treatment is most successful. The regimen used and pioneered by Dr. Vladimir Zelenko with his New York COVID-19 patients has been HCQ 200 mg BID, zinc sulphate 220 mg QD and azithromycin 500 mg QD, for 5 days each.[290] Dr. Zelenko has shared this information freely with the public as well as the medical community, and as of this writing, his clinical team has treated over 3000 COVID-19 patients, and 99.3% of their high risk COVID-19 patients have survived.

Dr. Zelenko found that nebulizing hydroxychloroquine was well tolerated and showed faster improvement, within one hour after use, in breathing in COVID-19 infected patients. His protocol is 6 ml (25 mg HCQ per ml) per nebulizer session (15 minutes). These were prescribed as 150 mg HCQ (2 ampules of 3 ml of HCQ each, at 25 mg / ml.) This is administered over 15 minutes via nebulizer. In comparison, the improvement that he observed with oral dosing of HCQ tablets was 80 hours. 95% of COVID-19 patients with pulmonary symptoms responded to this treatment. [291]

A retrospective study of 3,737 COVID-19 patients treated with HCQ and azithromycin showed early treatment correlated to significantly better clinical outcome, as well as faster reduction in viral burden. Risk of death was 59% lower in the treatment group.[292]

The combination of HCQ, azithromycin and zinc has shown outstanding results in resolving COVID-19. Of 405 COVID-19 patients, whose symptoms had been worse than "mild," treated in this study, only six were hospitalized, and two died.[293]

A pre-exposure prophylaxis study involved 4,239 very high risk healthcare workers, including doctors and nurses, in a hospital with up to 500 COVID-19 patients at a time. 1% of the healthcare workers were infected, and all of those recovered.[294] There were 8 mild symptomatic cases and no deaths. It was notable that all of the healthcare workers in the study worked with COVID-19 patients.[295]

In another retrospective case-control study of healthcare workers in India, cohorts were divided based on positive or negative PCR results. An inverse association was found between the number of HCQ doses consumed and the risk of positive COVID-19 test results.[296]

In a retrospective study of 518 patients receiving HCQ, zinc and azithromycin, the risk of death was found to be 79.4% lower in the treatment group than the control group, and the risk of hospitalization was found to be 81.6% lower.[297]

In this retrospective case series, the odds of hospitalization of those treated with HCQ, azithromycin and zinc were 84% less than the untreated group. Of 141 patients in the treated group, only one died.[298]

In this study of 3,473 patients there was a 24% reduced risk of in-hospital mortality.[299]

In August 2020, which was somewhat early in the COVID-19 era, virologist Steven Hatfill wrote of hydroxychloroquine:

"There are now 53 studies that show positive results of hydroxychloroquine in COVID infections. There are 14 global studies that show neutral or negative results – and 10 of them were of patients in very late stages of COVID-19, where no antiviral drug can be expected to have much effect. Of the remaining four studies, two come from the same University of Minnesota author. The author of two are from the faulty Brazil paper, which should be retracted, and the fake Lancet paper, which was." [300]

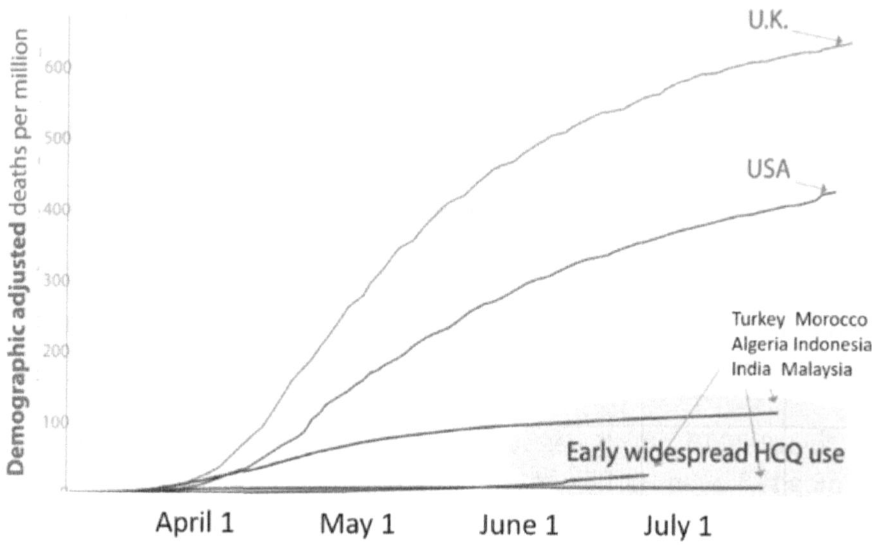

Graph © Steven Hatfill.[301]

Yale epidemiology professor Harvey Risch, a highly respected scientist with over 300 published peer-reviewed studies and 39,779 citations on Google Scholar, writes of the contrast between the successful clinical use of HCQ and zinc on the one hand, and its suppression by governments and industry on the other:

"I am fighting for a treatment that the data fully support but which, for reasons having nothing to do with a correct understanding of the science, has been pushed to the sidelines. As a result, tens of thousands of patients with COVID-19 are dying unnecessarily. Fortunately, the situation can be reversed easily and quickly." [302]

Dr. Risch adds that "US cumulative deaths through July 15, 2020 are 140,000. Had we permitted HCQ use liberally, we would have saved half, 70,000, and it is very possible we could have saved 3/4, or 105,000."

How effective is HCQ used against COVID-19 ? A real-time meta-analysis of 219 studies from around the world of hydroxychloroquine used for COVID-19 included results from 187,579 patients. It answers that question of how effective HCQ is against COVID-19:

> ***"HCQ is effective for COVID-19. The probability that an ineffective treatment generated results as positive as the 219 studies to date is estimated to be 1 in 327 quadrillion (p = 0.0000000000000000031).***
> ***And:***
> ***"92% of Randomized Controlled Trials (RCTs) for early, pre-exposure prophylaxis or post-exposure prophylaxis treatment report positive effects. The probability of this happening for an ineffective treatment is 0.0032."***
> ***And***
> ***"Studies from North America are 3.4 times more likely to report negative results than studies from the rest of the world combined, p = 0.00000046.***[303]

This meta-analysis should be read and studied by anyone who has ever feared COVID-19.

A database of all hydroxychloroquine / COVID-19 studies to date as of this writing, includes 273 studies, with 200 of them peer-reviewed. 221 of these studies compare treatment and control groups. Those who compile the database find that the studies are consistent in showing that "early treatment consistently shows positive effects."[304]

* * *

There are other zinc ionophores that are also being used together with zinc against COVID-19.

Zinc and quercitin vs COVID-19

Quercitin is a flavonoid, which is a resilient plant-derived antioxidant. It was shown in this study to have ionophoric action with zinc in mouse studies.[305]

Quercitin has also shown anti-viral effect against RNA virus Influenza A, H1N1 and H3N2. This in vitro study showed that quercitin bound to viral proteins and that it caused significant inhibition on viral protein synthesis in a dose-dependent way.[306]

Zinc and EGCG vs COVID-19

Epigallocatechin-gallate (EGCG) has been found in the same study as above to have zinc ionophoric activity. [307]

This extract from the common household beverage green tea was also found to have antiviral mechanisms apart from its ability to move zinc into a cell, and has shown activity against a wide variety of viruses, including RNA viruses. EGCG inhibits virus attachment and entry into cells. It does this by interference with viral proteins. It also inhibits RNA synthesis by viral RNA polymerase. These antiviral mechanisms of EGCG are summarized in this paper.[308] Roasting green tea converts EGCG to different molecules, which may result in different effects from black tea than from green tea.

Ivermectin sends COVID to lockdown

Ivermectin is on the WHO List of Essential Medicines and is approved by the FDA. This well-tolerated but potent anti-parasitic medicine has been prescribed billions of times in its 36-year history against a wide range of parasites. It is a drug in the avermectin family, so named because those compounds are produced by the soil organism *Streptomyces avermitilis.* It has also been studied and used against a wide range of viruses especially over the last decade, and there is evidence of potent antiviral effects against Influenza A and over a dozen other viruses tested.[309]

In a meta-analysis of 49 trials of ivermectin versus COVID-19 in humans, 100% of these have shown positive results. Studies were from all continents except Antarctica. Considered individually, 24 of those studies were found to be statistically significant. Over the 49 studies in meta-analysis, pooled effects showed 80% reduced infections, and prophylactic use showed 89% improvement, and 76% lower mortality. Of those studies in the meta-analysis that were peer-reviewed, overall improvement in early treatment was found to be 83% (74% in randomized controlled trials), and 92% of those in which ivermectin was used prophylactically showed improvement (91% in randomized controlled trials).

Mortality from COVID-19 over all time periods of delay in treatment was 76% improved over controls (69% in randomized controlled trials), whereas mortality was improved 84% in early treatment of COVID-19 (82% in randomized controlled trials). Forty studies were excluded from the meta-analysis for complicating factors or insufficient detail reported, and these also showed 100% positive results.

It is estimated that the likelihood of an ineffective treatment showing such positive results as the above results in the 49 studies in the meta-analysis to date is exceedingly small. That probability is estimated to be 1 in 563 trillion.[310] The overall results of the meta-analysis were not only found to be "overwhelmingly positive," but also "very consistent, and very insensitive to potential selection criteria, effect extraction rules, and/or bias evaluation."

The first clinical trial of ivermectin in COVID-19 patients was an observational study in four Florida hospitals from March to May 2020. Even in patients with severe pulmonary involvement, mortality was 38.8% in the treatment group vs 80.7% in controls, and this group showed the strongest mortality difference from controls, which raised the possibility of ivermectin also being available as a salvage or rescue treatment.[311]

In a randomized controlled trial, patients given ivermectin were 8 times more likely to be medically released than those in the placebo group. This was even though the average age and number of co-morbidities were later found to be somewhat higher in the experimental group than in the control group.[312]

The African continent has had remarkably low incidence of COVID-19, particularly equatorial African countries. It may be helpful to look at African countries where ivermectin has been used commonly for decades against the onchocerciasis that it has been prescribed for, to observe population-wide effects. In this population comparison, risk of COVID-19 death was found to be 88.2% lower and mortality 85.7% lower in 31 countries where onchocerciasis is endemic and ivermectin is commonly used than in 22 countries where neither is the case, even though the latter group of countries has a higher life expectancy, 66 years vs 61 years.[313]

Ivermectin, for all its power against viruses, is among the safest of medicines that are in long-term and widespread use.[314] There are no known serious drug-related adverse events.[315] Again, it is commonly taken by the populations of 31 African countries for effect against endemic parasites. Dosing has been given as a single annual dose of 150 mcg/kg against filariasis. There have been very few serious adverse events reported over more than 30 years of use. 37 of approximately 14,000 patients treated in Ghana had symptomatic posture hypotension, associated with fainting or sweating or tachycardia. These were treated with corticosteroids.[316] This Lancet study determined its safety in pregnant women, and the risk of fetal damage was not greater than in control women's fetuses.[317]

However, despite this safety data going back 3 decades, the US FDA has alleged, "Any use of ivermectin for the prevention or treatment of COVID-19 should be avoided as its benefits and safety for these purposes have not been established." The FDA offered no supporting evidence for their claim.[318] One concerning risk is that ivermectin is sold over the counter for veterinary use, and if people feel desperate to use it to ward off COVID-19, they might break off too large a piece from a large horse pill. For this reason, it is much better to consult a healthcare provider for ivermectin use and dosing. To further enhance safety, liposomal ivermectin carriers have been developed. When these were used against Dengue fever, cytotoxicity was reduced up to 5 times, absorption was faster and *in vivo* efficacy was improved.[319]

Despite the spectacular worldwide effect profile, of excellent effect against COVID-19, with 0.26% observed minor side effects, and its use across several continents, ivermectin is widely shunned and ignored in western Europe and in the US. Here is a brief synopsis of how that came to be.

Ivermectin was invented in Japan in 1975 as an anti-parasitic drug by Satoshi Omura, a Kitasato University professor emeritus, which earned Dr. Omura the Nobel Prize in Biochemistry. Ivermectin turned out to be quite effective against a broad spectrum of parasites. The drug was so effective in eliminating a range of parasitic infections, and at very low cost, about $0.10 US, that 3.7 billion doses have been delivered to much of the world's population since its invention.[320]

A cell culture study in April 2020 showed a 5000 times reduction in SARS-CoV-2 from one dose over 48 hours, compared to control samples.[321] Several Latin American countries, Egypt and India soon began to use it for COVID-19, and then South Africa and several European countries as well. However, resistance remained strong in the US and western Europe, following the vocal disapproval of The World Health Organization (WHO), The US National Institutes of Health (NIH), the US Food and Drug Administration (FDA) and the European Medicine Agency (EMA). These agencies all expressed disapproval of ivermectin for use with COVID-19 patients. Even after more than 20 randomized controlled clinical trials showed promising effect without adverse reactions, many western countries have still not adopted its use.

Social media companies censored ivermectin research. Even when the WHO commissioned and reported a meta-analysis of ivermectin, it was censored by YouTube. Only negative commentaries were permitted in western media.[322]

How does ivermectin send SARS-CoV-2 to lockdown? There are a number of mechanisms by which components of SARS-CoV-2 need to stay mobile and active in order to replicate, and thus to spread throughout the human body. It turns out that ivermectin binds several of these, which inactivates the virus. Let's look at exactly what happens to bind or to lock down SARS-CoV-2.

RNA-dependent RNA-polymerase (RdRp) is one of the main enzymes used by SARS-CoV-2 to achieve RNA replication. It is required for viral genome replication, and therefore it is helpful if a nutrient or drug can act on it as an obstacle in some way. 173 drugs were tested in this study for their ability to bind RdRp (making it unavailable or inactive), including two examined in this book, hydroxychloroquine and vitamin C, although vitamin C was also found to have relatively high binding energy for RdRp in this study. Of all the drugs tested, ivermectin was found to bind RdRp with higher binding any energy than any other drug.[323]

One strategy against SARS-CoV-2, as well as other endemic and pandemic RNA viruses, has been to interfere with transport of viruses into a host cell's nucleus. Ivermectin has been shown to accomplish this by binding, destabilizing and inhibiting the protein IMP alpha/beta1. When this protein is inhibited, viruses are unable to enter a cell's nucleus, and therefore unable to replicate. Decreased infection results. IMP alpha/beta 1 has been inhibited in SARS-CoV-2 entry into nuclei by ivermectin.[324] Previously, it has been observed that ivermectin inhibited that same protein from entry of other RNA viruses, giving it a broad-spectrum antiviral effect.[325] [326] [327]

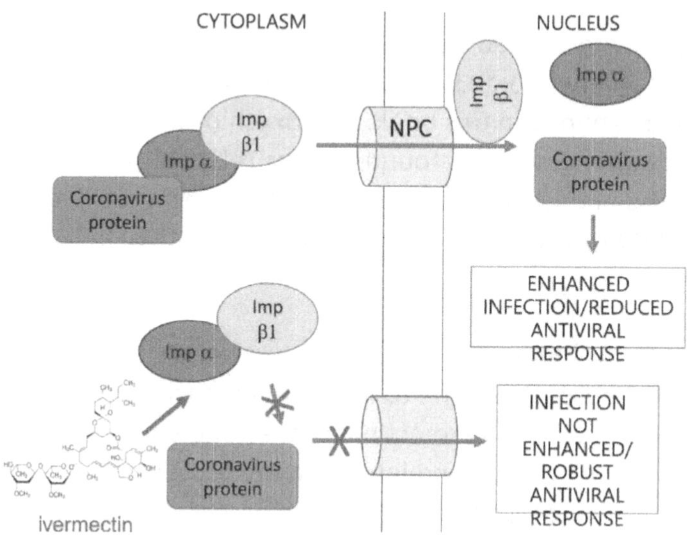

Figure © L Caly, J Druce, et al., Endnote 321.

It turns out that ivermectin not only binds tightly to RdRp on SARS-CoV-2, and IMP alpha/beta1; it also strongly binds the spike protein on SARS-CoV-2. This particular spike protein is trimeric, meaning it has 3 subunits which vary in amino acid sequences or other ways. It was observed that ivermectin binds all three of the SARS-CoV-2 subunits, both the structural S2 subunit, as well as both of the two functional S1 subunits.[328] This binding of all 3 subunits of the trimeric spike protein may be considered a trifecta of fortunate results of ivermectin in favor of the human host and in opposition to the SARS-CoV-2 virus.

Ivermectin has different mechanisms against parasites, already a miraculous healing drug for that use alone through much of the world's population. However, now that we learn of its tremendous effect in binding both RdRp and all three trimers of the spike protein of SARS-CoV-2, we are certainly fortunate to have this medicine in our arsenal against COVID-19. It is inexpensive, and full COVID-19 treatment of an individual, from first dose till last needed can be less than one US dollar. Ivermectin is therefore available to even the poorest communities in the world. Ivermectin is being compared to the discovery of penicillin in its enormous impact, and perhaps was one of the greatest discoveries of the 20th century.[329] The fact that this tremendously effective, safe and low-cost antiviral drug is not as thoroughly known to the world as penicillin is a chasm of inexcusable and deadly ignorance that the COVID era is giving the world an opportunity to correct.

Part III: What does not work against COVID

"They were sure about lockdowns.
They were wrong.
They were sure about closing schools.
They were wrong.
They were sure about masks.
They were wrong.
Now they're so sure about vaccines – vaccines using totally new biotechnology – they want to mandate them.
What could go wrong?"

Alex Berenson
Journalist and a leading spokesperson for "Team Reality"

For a year, those of us who are familiar with world history and / or basic mathematics and / or a medical school education, especially those of us who stayed awake in immunology and medical history classes have been reaching out to our fellow frightened humans and urging them to consider that the widely proposed and adopted cures for COVID would likely turn out to be much worse than the disease itself. We predicted widespread and enduring morbidity and mortality from governments' public health measures, and so far we have unfortunately been proven correct. Lockdowns did not save lives, and masks only worsened COVID-19. The proof is in the following pages.

But our warnings were largely to no avail, as Team Reality has had nearly all of our microphones turned off. Big Tech and social media censorship silenced many of us, even those of us, myself included, who posted only data from peer-reviewed medical journals, government webpages and mainstream news sources. I was suspended from Twitter 5 times, four times for posting peer-reviewed research and once for a US government webpage, which showed the hazards of masks. When those of us in Team Reality presented evidence that challenged the official narrative beyond a certain point, we were censored, and we in Team Reality remain with much smaller reach than Public Health "experts." Even Dr. Zelenko, who showed the world how to defeat COVID, including very clearly on social media, has been suspended from Twitter for several months as of this writing.

Yet those experts turned out to be wrong, about everything related to COVID. Let's see in the following chapters how the draconian actions of our governments failed to reduce the virus, and failed in so many other ways that injured people's most precious possessions: our contact with loved ones, our childrens' education, our jobs and livelihoods, and our essential civil liberties.

PDMJ

Lockdowns failed to reduce deaths in the US:

Total deaths declined more, from previous years, in free states than in lockdown states in spring 2020.

June 12, 2020.
Completed peer-review and revised, December 4, 2020
Colleen Huber, NMD[iii]
https://pdmj.org/papers/lockdowns_failed_to_reduce_deaths_in_the_us/

Abstract

A control group and an experimental group for a single variable in a scientific experiment are not often provided by political events. All except six US states instituted lockdowns in the spring of 2020. This paper compares mortality data from those six states, herein "free states," with their immediate neighbors, "locked states," and with all of the 44 locked states. Five weeks of mortality data during the gradual easing of lockdown in most US states during the spring of 2020 show a consistent history among those weeks with regard to the following: Free states had a lower percentage than locked states of

[iii] Colleen Huber, NMD is a Naturopathic Medical Doctor and Naturopathic Oncologist (FNORI), writing on topics of masks, COVID-19, cancer and nutrition.

total deaths from all causes in these weeks in 2020, compared to the same weeks for each of the states in the years 2017 to 2019.

Each free state had fewer deaths in comparison to its own record of recent years. Locked states averaged more deaths compared to their own records of recent years. This difference holds for both of the following comparisons: free vs locked states that are immediately surrounding free states, as well as free states compared to the average results of all locked states in the US.

Introduction

US Centers for Disease Control and Prevention (CDC) data from weeks ending May 15, 2020 through June 12, 2020 show consistency over each of those five weeks in the following data.

Five US states: Arkansas, Iowa, Nebraska, North Dakota and South Dakota, did not lock down, and submitted mortality data to the CDC. These states are the control group, herein "free states" in the mass human experiment of society-wide lockdown in the spring of 2020.

There are other states that have special situations. Wyoming also did not lock down, but the CDC had not posted complete mortality data for Wyoming until June 10, 2020, so I exclude Wyoming in most of the following weeks; however, June 12, 2020 data for Wyoming is included in the June 12, 2020 table (Table 5). Also, Utah and Oklahoma did not impose lockdown at the state level; however, lockdown was imposed in their most populous jurisdictions, so I group Utah and Oklahoma with the locked states. USA Today lists states that locked down, opened up and the dates for each.[330] That article shows that almost all states locked down during the last 10 days of March, 2020. Most states began re-opening during the first three weeks of

May, 2020. The CDC shows peak COVID-19 deaths as mid-April in this table.[331]

For comparison with the five free states, I also look at CDC mortality data of the immediately neighboring states, with which the free states share long borders. These are respectively, Mississippi, Louisiana, Missouri, Oklahoma, Minnesota, Wisconsin, Illinois, Kansas, Colorado and Montana. These are the states in the immediately surrounding experimental group, herein "locked states." Many of these states have comparable population density with their neighboring free states, varying more in density from urban to rural areas within states than from interstate comparisons of density.

This paper will examine CDC data to determine whether reduction in deaths happened in US states that locked down.

Lockdowns were imposed by many jurisdictions for the stated purpose of limiting local and long-distance travel, activities involving human interaction, education, religious congregation and sports events, as well as commerce of individuals and certain types of businesses, for the stated goal of limiting COVID-19 incidence and mortality. Children throughout the US have been kept out of classrooms through most of 2020, and ill patients have been kept away from medical treatment. It was widely hoped this would work. However, outside of the US, it was found that mortality actually increased steeply closely following lockdowns.[332] Also, it was found that in Europe, "no lives were saved" by lockdown.[333] In an early analysis in the US also, it was not found that lives were saved by shutdown.[334] Those last two analyses were relatively early, 4/24 and 4/26/20 respectively, before it was clear that COVID-19 incidence, hospitalizations and deaths had peaked. As of this writing in December 2020, peak COVID-19 hospitalizations and deaths occurred the week of April 18, 2020 in the US as is seen in Graph 1 below.

Graph 1

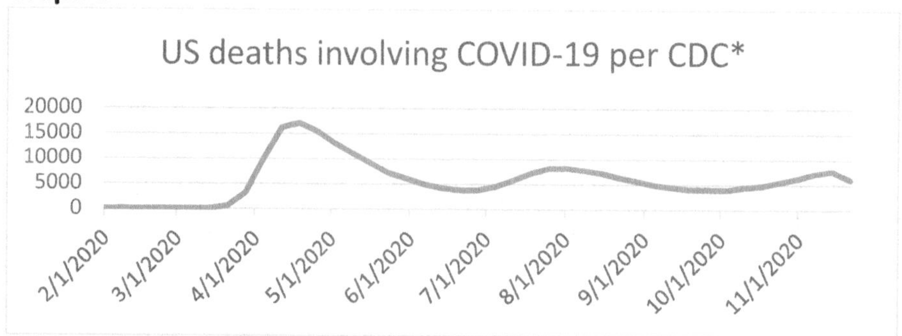

*From column "All deaths involving COVID-19"
https://www.cdc.gov/nchs/nvss/vsrr/covid19/index.htm

This study is likewise of a limited time frame, the five weeks of the decline of lockdown, and the advent of re-opening. Through the five weeks of this study, there is stark and consistent contrast of mortality in free vs. locked states.

Methods

In this study, I examine whether lockdowns succeeded in reducing total deaths, and whether that data is consistent over the five weeks immediately following when most lockdowns through the US began to ease. In order to answer the question of whether lockdowns succeeded in reducing mortality, it is most helpful to look at all deaths, because total deaths are more precisely enumerated than deaths from any specific cause, due to common multiple co-morbidities.

I chose to examine total deaths rather than COVID-19 deaths in this study for a number of additional reasons, including the following:

1) The very questionable applicability of the manufacturing technique, the reverse-transcriptase / polymerase chain

reaction (PCR "test"), now used throughout the world as a test for presence of an infectious agent; and

2) The 80% and higher reported false positive rate of this "test" in the diagnosis of COVID-19, [335] leading to a forever unknowable true number of total COVID-19 deaths; and
3) The arbitrary number of iterations of this "test" that have been selected to produce a positive result[336]; and
4) Instructions given to physicians by the CDC to code cases as COVID-19 deaths including presumptively[337]; and
5) Controversy regarding higher Medicare reimbursement for COVID-19 patients ($13,000)[338] than for flu patients ($5,000), which may have skewed reported cause of death on death certificates; and
6) The possibility that there may be emergency aid incentives and/or political influences in altering the true number of deaths from COVID-19; and
7) If COVID-19 is genuinely the deadly pandemic that it is widely thought to be, then total deaths in any jurisdiction would be greater during the period of its peak incidence and closely following weeks. It is not possible to have a deadly pandemic rage through a population without increasing the total number of all-cause deaths over the weeks of its peak incidence. Therefore, if deaths are not significantly increased above previous years for a given region, then there has been no pandemic, nor even an epidemic there. It is possible that lockdowns decreased numbers of fatal motor vehicle accidents, even with fewer vehicles and higher speeds, but increased numbers of suicide and substance abuse deaths have been recorded. This is a complex topic for examination elsewhere.

Therefore, it is most useful and most accurate to look at total deaths in each state, both in free states, the control group, as well as in locked states, the experimental group.

The CDC shows a percentage of deaths in each state compared with the same week in previous years. This percentage for each is described by the CDC as follows: "Percent of expected deaths is the number of deaths for all causes for this week in 2020 compared to the average number across the same week in 2017-2019."[339]

The CDC compares each of the states, free and locked, to their own mortality history from 2017 through 2019. I then compare those two groups to each other. The CDC tables from which the numbers in this study were derived are screen-printed in this endnote. [340] These tables are from Friday, May 15, 2020, Friday, May 22, 2020, Friday, May 29, 2020, Friday, June 5, 2020 and Friday, June 12, 2020.

The above-mentioned CDC tables are the entire source from which all calculated data in this paper is derived. No other source is used, and all derived data may be verified by the reader with a simple calculator.

The following five tables show a comparison of free vs locked states, regarding each state's mortality for that week as a percentage of the same week in the years 2017 to 2019. These are shown for each of the last five weeks. The tables show comparison of % expected deaths of the total of the free states with the total of their neighboring locked states, control group vs experimental group, over each of those weeks.

Table 1: Week ending 5/15/2020

A	B	C	D	E
	5/15/2020 Percent of expected deaths for this week wrt prior years		Percent of expected deaths for this week wrt prior years	
Free states	(from CDC table)	Neighboring locked states	(from CDC table)	
AR	96	MS	102	
IA	96	LA	103	
NE	89	MO	93	
ND	83	OK	85	
SD	90	MN	103	
		WI	103	
		IL	109	
		KS	97	
		CO	109	
		MT	88	
Average	90.8	Average	99.2	
		Average factor by which % of all expected deaths are higher in locked states than in free states	(average of Col. D / Col. B)	1.09

Table 2: Week ending 5/22/2020

A	B	C	D	E
	5/22/2020 Percent of expected deaths for this week wrt prior years		Percent of expected deaths for this week wrt prior years	
Free states	(from CDC table)	Neighboring locked states	(from CDC table)	
AR	98	MS	101	
IA	97	LA	105	
NE	95	MO	95	
ND	83	OK	85	
SD	93	MN	104	
		WI	105	
		IL	112	
		KS	97	
		CO	111	
		MT	90	
Average	93.2	Average	100.5	
		Average factor by which % of all expected deaths are higher in locked states than in free states	(average of Col. D / Col. B)	1.08

Table 3: Week ending 5/29/2020

A	B	C	D	E
	5/29/2020			
	Percent of		Percent of	
	expected		expected	
	deaths for		deaths for	
	this week		this week	
	wrt prior years		wrt prior years	
Free		Neighboring		
states	(from CDC table)	locked states	(from CDC table)	
AR	96	MS	104	
IA	98	LA	105	
NE	96	MO	94	
ND	79	OK	84	
SD	91	MN	104	
		WI	102	
		IL	112	
		KS	97	
		CO	111	
		MT	90	
Average	92.0	Average	100.3	
		Average factor by which	(average	1.09
		% of all expected deaths	of	
		are higher	Col. D / Col. B)	
		in locked states		
		than in free states		

Table 4: Week ending 6/5/2020

A	B	C	D	E
	6/5/2020			
	Percent of		Percent of	
	expected		expected	
	deaths for		deaths for	
	this week		this week	
	wrt prior years		wrt prior years	
Free		Neighboring		
states	(from CDC table)	locked states	(from CDC table)	
AR	97	MS	105	
IA	99	LA	107	
NE	94	MO	96	
ND	79	OK	90	
SD	92	MN	105	
		WI	103	
		IL	114	
		KS	98	
		CO	111	
		MT	92	
Average	92.2	Average	102.1	
		Average factor by which	(average	1.11
		% of all expected deaths	of	
		are higher	Col. D / Col. B)	
		in locked states		
		than in free states		

Table 5: Week ending 6/12/2020

A	B	C	D	E
	6/12/2020 Percent of expected deaths for this week wrt prior years		Percent of expected deaths for this week wrt prior years	
Free states	(from CDC table)	Neighboring locked states	(from CDC table)	
AR	96	MS	104	
IA	98	LA	107	
NE	95	MO	95	
ND	79	OK	91	
SD	92	MN	103	
WY	99	WI	102	
		IL	113	
		KS	96	
		CO	109	
		MT	93	
		ID	97	
Average	93.2	Average	**100.9**	
		Average factor by which % of all expected deaths are higher in locked states than in free states	(average of Col. D / Col. B)	**1.08**

From the above tables, over the last five weeks of easing of lockdowns, the average factor by which the percentage of all expected deaths are higher in locked states as a group than in free states as a group has stayed fairly consistent, between 1.08 and 1.11.

The locked states as a group averaged 8% to 11% higher percentage of deaths than the free states did over their own previous years' records. This is expressed in the following graph showing locked vs free states vs all states, from tables in Endnote 11.

Graph 2

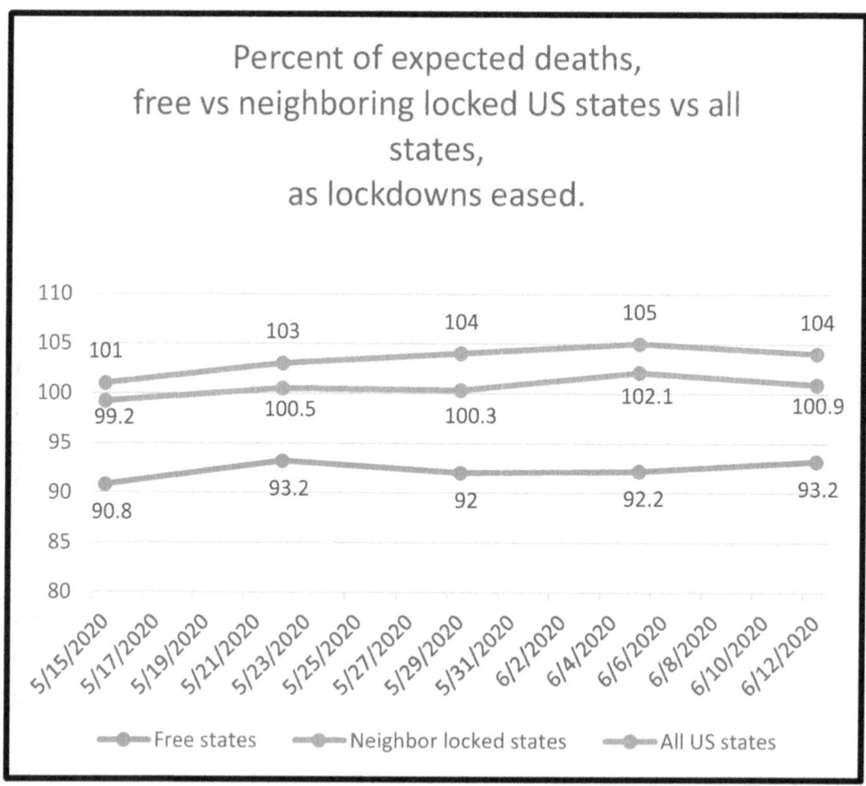

As lockdowns ease, and conditions in formerly locked vs free states begin to resemble their own previous years' conditions, these different percentages would be expected to gradually converge toward 100% for each state, and Graph 2 suggests that this had already begun to happen toward the end of the five weeks observed.

Finally, let's compare the 6 free states with 44 locked states from June 12, 2020 (the day of this preprint writing) CDC data (now including Wyoming, because June 10, 2020, is the first date of mortality data for Wyoming in the CDC tables.) That comparison is in Tables 6a and 6b, divided into two tables only because of the long list of 44 states, listed alphabetically.

Table 6a: Week ending 6/12/2020, all states, part 1 of 2

A	B	C	D
	ALL STATES		
	6/12/2020		
	Percent of expected deaths for this week wrt prior years		Percent of expected deaths for this week wrt prior years
Free states	(from CDC table)	Locked states	(from CDC table)
AR	96	AL	97
IA	98	AK	87
NE	95	AZ	105
ND	79	CA	101
SD	92	CO	109
WY	99	CT	72
		DC	115
		DE	102
		FL	101
		GA	99
		HI	95
		ID	97
		IL	113
		IN	103
		KS	96
		KY	91
		LA	107
		ME	98
		MD	115
		MA	127
		MI	111

Table 6b: Week ending 6/12/2020, all states, part 2 of 2

A	B	C	D	E
		MN	103	
		MS	104	
		MO	95	
		MT	93	
		NV	99	
		NH	102	
		NJ	151	
		NM	96	
		NY except NYC	128	
		NYC	220	
		NC	73	
		OH	94	
		OK	91	
		OR	94	
		PA	93	
		RI	102	
		SC	104	
		TN	97	
		TX	98	
		UT	98	
		VT	102	
		VA	104	
		WA	100	
		WV	80	
		WI	102	
Average	93.2	Average	**103.6**	
		Average factor by which % of all expected deaths are higher in locked states than in free states	(average of Col. D / Col. B)	**1.11**

* The CDC counts New York City data separately from the rest of New York State. This was considered in the average, as if New York City were a different state. The CDC also includes data from Washington, DC. Therefore, there are 6 states on the left, and 44 states plus two cities, NYC and DC, on the right.

Now it can be seen that not only comparing neighboring states, free vs locked, but also looking at the entire United States, there is a consistent pattern: Free states show fewer than expected deaths during this week than previous years at this time. Moreover, free states had a distinct survival advantage, and significantly lower mortality than locked states, when each state is compared with its own previous record. The factor by which locked states' mortality change (as percent of expected) exceeded free states' mortality change (as percent of expected) was consistently positive and by a factor of 1.08 to 1.11.

Conclusion

Because the free states did not have increased deaths from their data in previous years, but their neighboring locked states, with similar population density, did average increased deaths over the free states from their data in previous years, by a factor that stayed within the narrow range of 1.08 to 1.11 through the five weeks that included both peak COVID-19 mortality and included the end of, and the easing of lockdown, it can be concluded therefore with certainty that lockdown did not reduce deaths in the US.

In fact, free states had decreased deaths from their data in previous years, but locked states on average did not have decreased deaths from their data in previous years. This establishes with certainty that lockdown did not reduce deaths. How is this conclusion certain? Because if a popular hypothesis is that A caused B (lockdowns caused reduced deaths), but it then becomes clear that B never happened, then we can confidently surmise that A definitely did not cause B. Causation is very hard to prove, but lack of causation is very easy to prove, particularly when the effect never happened. We can be certain that A did not cause B, if we see that B never happened at all. Lockdown did happen in most US states, including the states surrounding the free states, which I examined. However, deaths were not reduced in those locked states, neither in comparison to their own historical mortality data on average, nor in comparison to their free neighbors. Total deaths from all causes were not reduced in the locked states, as is seen in the above data.

This paper examined CDC data to determine whether reduction in deaths happened in lockdown states. That did not happen; therefore, there is nothing, including lockdowns, that has caused it to happen.

The conclusion and its supporting data impact future assessments of whether lockdown was an optimal strategy of state governments. A failure of lockdowns to reduce deaths must in the future be considered when weighed against the considerable damage, including political, economic, humanitarian, social and psychological damage and even deaths, caused directly by lockdowns. Society's response to the phenomenon of COVID-19 led to the loss of 30 million to 40 million jobs in the US alone.[341] The US unemployment rate rose to 14.7%. [342] Unemployment's adverse effects are known to reverberate through families and communities and business sectors, and must be considered in the future, if lockdown is ever proposed again. The consistently worse (by 8 to 11%) mortality results that I showed in locked states over free states likely reflect the life-threatening consequences of mass unemployment. Civil liberties concerns are also paramount to those who value those liberties perhaps as highly as their own lives, aware of wars throughout American history and world history that were fought in defense of or to establish the same. Those liberties were challenged, curtailed and violated to various degrees throughout the US, as a consequence of lockdowns. Therefore, lockdowns had historic and far-reaching social, political and economic effects, but they did not reduce deaths, and therefore cannot be justified now or in the future. The timeframe of this study is limited, however, and a more thorough assessment of lockdown impact on mortality would be obtained by a study of more weeks than the five examined herein.

Free states continue survival advantage over locked states after most lockdowns ease

This June 26, 2020 update of the previous paper was not submitted for peer review. It is an update of the June 12, 2020 paper, "Lockdowns failed to reduce deaths in the US: Total deaths declined more, from previous years, in free states than in lockdown states."

Abstract

This paper is updated June 29, 2020, showing seven weeks of mortality data during and following the gradual easing of lockdown in most US states during the spring of 2020. There is a consistent history among those weeks with regard to the following: States without lockdown, herein "free states," have had a lower percentage than states with lockdown, herein "locked states," of total deaths from all causes in these weeks in 2020, compared to the same weeks for each of the states in the years 2017 to 2019.

Each free state had fewer deaths in comparison to its own record of recent years. Locked states averaged more deaths compared to their own records of recent years.

These are holding true even after most lockdowns have eased or ended.

This difference holds for both of the following comparisons: free vs locked states that are immediately surrounding free states, as well as free states compared to the average results of all locked states in the US.

Introduction

US Centers for Disease Control and Prevention (CDC) data from weeks ending May 15, 2020 through June 26, 2020 show consistency over each of those seven weeks in the following data.

Five US states: Arkansas, Iowa, Nebraska, North Dakota and South Dakota, did not lock down, and submitted mortality data to the CDC. These states are the control group, herein "free states" in the mass human experiment of society-wide lockdown in the spring of 2020.

There are other states that have special situations. Wyoming also did not lock down, but the CDC had not posted complete mortality data for Wyoming until June 10, 2020, so I exclude Wyoming in most of the following weeks; however, June 12 through 26, 2020 data for Wyoming is included in the June 12 through 26, 2020 tables (Table 5-7). Also, Utah and Oklahoma did not impose lockdown at the state level; however, lockdown was imposed in their most populous jurisdictions, so I group Utah and Oklahoma with the locked states. USA Today lists states that locked down, opened up and the dates for each.[343] That article shows that almost all states locked down during the last 10 days of March, 2020. Most states began re-opening during the first three weeks of May, 2020. The CDC shows peak COVID-19 deaths as occurring in mid-April 2020 in this table.[344]

For comparison with the five free states, I also look at CDC mortality data of the immediately neighboring states, with which the free states share long borders. These are respectively, Mississippi, Louisiana, Missouri, Oklahoma, Minnesota, Wisconsin, Illinois, Kansas, Colorado and Montana. These are the states in the immediately surrounding experimental group, herein "locked states."

This paper will examine CDC data to determine whether reduction in deaths happened in US states that locked down.

Lockdowns were imposed by many jurisdictions for the stated purpose of limiting movement, activities and commerce of individuals and businesses, for the goal of limiting COVID-19 incidence and mortality. It was widely hoped this would work for that purpose. However, outside of the US, it was found that mortality actually increased steeply closely following lockdowns.[345] Also, it was found that in Europe, "no lives were saved" by lockdown.[346] In an early analysis in the US also, it was not found that lives were saved by shutdown.[347] Those last two analyses were relatively early, 4/24 and 4/26/20 respectively, before it was clear that COVID-19 incidence, hospitalizations and deaths had peaked.

This study is likewise of a limited time frame, the seven weeks of the decline of lockdown, the American perestroika, one might say, of re-opening. Through the seven weeks of this study there is stark and consistent contrast of mortality in free vs. locked states.

Table 6: Week ending 6/19/2020

A	B	C	D	E
	6/19/2020 Percent of expected deaths for this week wrt prior years		Percent of expected deaths for this week wrt prior years	
Free states	(from CDC table)	Neighboring locked states	(from CDC table)	
AR	97	MS	107	
IA	99	LA	108	
NE	98	MO	97	
ND	81	OK	92	
SD	93	MN	107	
WY	101	WI	104	
		IL	116	
		KS	98	
		CO	111	
		MT	96	
		ID	99	
Average	94.8	Average	103.2	
		Average factor by which % of all expected deaths are higher in locked states than in free states	(average of Col. D / Col. B)	1.09

Table 7: Week ending 6/26/2020

A	B	C	D	E
	6/26/2020			
	Percent of		Percent of	
	expected		expected	
	deaths for		deaths for	
	this week		this week	
	wrt prior years		wrt prior years	
Free		Neighboring		
states	(from CDC table)	locked states	(from CDC table)	
AR	100	MS	107	
IA	100	LA	108	
NE	99	MO	97	
ND	79	OK	92	
SD	90	MN	107	
WY	100	WI	104	
		IL	116	
		KS	98	
		CO	111	
		MT	96	
		ID	99	
Average	94.7	Average	103.2	
		Average factor by which	(average	1.09
		% of all expected deaths	of	
		are higher	Col. D / Col. B)	
		in locked states		
		than in free states		

We see that over the last seven weeks of easing of lockdowns, the average factor by which the percentage of all expected deaths are higher in locked states as a group than in free states as a group has stayed fairly consistent, between 1.08 and 1.11.

The locked states as a group averaged an 8% to 11% higher percentage of deaths over their own previous years' records than the free states averaged. This is expressed in the following graph showing free states vs neighboring locked states vs all states, from tables in Endnote 11.

Graph 1

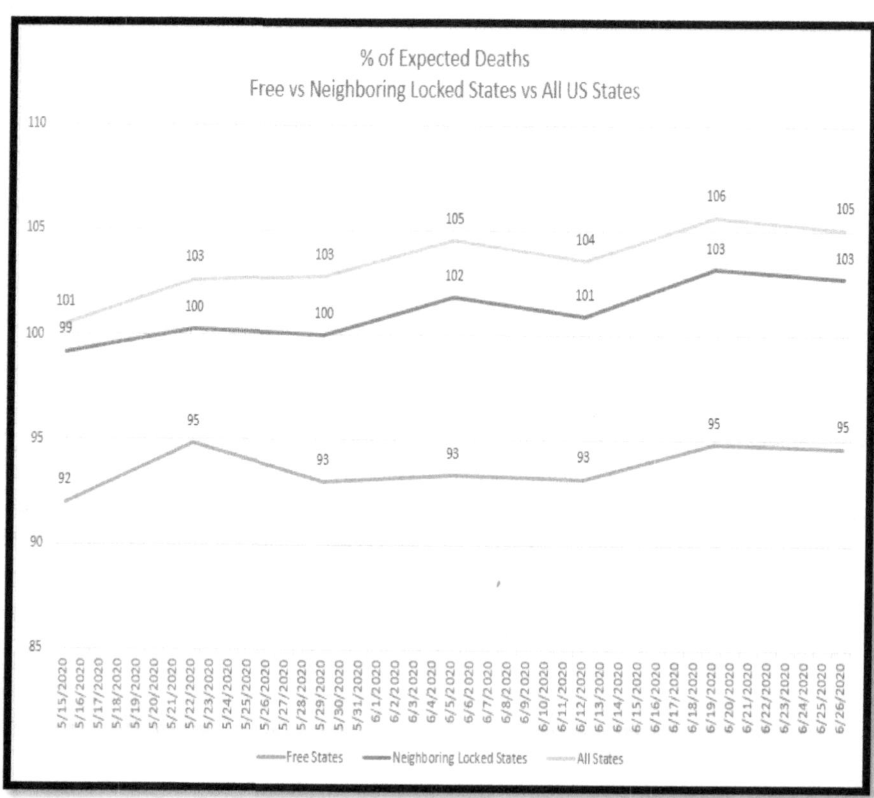

As lockdowns ease, and conditions in formerly locked vs free states begin to resemble their own previous years' conditions, these different percentages would be expected to gradually converge toward 100% for each state, and Graph 1 suggests that this has begun to happen, although it may be already too late in 2020 for those percentages to converge completely by the end of the year.

Finally, let's compare the 6 free states with 44 locked states from today's (the day of this writing) CDC data (now including Wyoming, because June 10, 2020, is the first date of mortality data for Wyoming in the CDC tables.) That comparison is in Tables 8a and 8b.

Table 3a: All 7 weeks, free states vs neighboring locked states

	5/15/20	5/22/20	5/29/20	6/5/20	6/12/20	6/19/20
Percent of expected deaths for this week with respect to prior years (from CDC table)						
FREE STATES						
AR	96	98	96	97	96	97
IA	96	97	98	99	98	99
NE	89	95	96	94	95	98
ND	83	83	79	79	79	81
SD	90	93	91	92	92	93
WY	98	103	98	99	99	101
Average	92	95	93	93	93	95
NEIGHBORING STATES						
MS	102	101	104	105	104	107
LA	103	105	105	107	107	108
MO	93	95	94	96	95	97
OK	85	85	84	90	91	92
MN	103	104	104	105	103	107
WI	103	105	102	103	102	104
IL	109	112	112	114	113	116
KS	97	97	97	98	96	98
CO	109	111	111	111	109	111
MT	88	90	90	92	93	96
ID	99	98	97	99	97	99
Average	99.2	100.3	100.0	101.8	100.9	103.2

	5/15/20	5/22/20	5/29/20	6/5/20	6/12/20	6/19/20	Average
Free States	92	95	93	93	93	95	94
Neighboring Locked States	99	100	100	102	101	103	101
All States	101	103	103	105	104	106	
Neighboring / free states							**1.08**

Table 3b: All weeks, all locked states
(on following page)

	05/15/ 2020	05/22/ 2020	05/29/ 2020	06/05/ 2020	06/12/ 2020	06/19/ 2020	06/26/ 2020

ALL LOCKED STATES, from CDC tables, % of expected deaths this week with respect to prior years

AL	95	95	96	98	97	99	99
AK	83	85	87	88	87	88	89
AZ	103	105	105	106	105	108	110
CA	99	100	101	102	101	103	103
CO	109	111	111	111	109	111	112
CT	37	48	51	66	72	78	85
DC	101	103	109	113	115	117	119
DE	93	96	100	100	102	103	98
FL	102	102	102	103	101	103	103
GA	95	97	98	99	99	101	100
HI	96	97	97	97	95	96	95
ID	99	98	97	99	97	99	99
IL	109	112	112	114	113	116	116
IN	102	102	104	105	103	104	100
KS	97	97	97	98	96	98	98
KY	88	90	89	91	91	92	94
LA	103	105	105	107	107	108	108
ME	101	101	100	101	98	101	100
MD	110	113	115	116	115	118	118
MA	125	128	127	130	127	129	128
MI	113	111	111	114	111	114	114
MN	103	104	104	105	103	107	106
MS	102	101	104	105	104	107	107
MO	93	95	94	96	95	97	97
MT	88	90	90	92	93	96	92
NV	98	100	100	100	99	101	100
NH	102	103	104	105	102	107	106
NJ	141	149	152	153	151	153	148
NM	93	93	95	96	96	96	96
NY, not NYC	129	130	131	131	128	130	129
NYC	236	236	232	228	220	219	213
NC	54	63	61	69	73	74	73
OH	90	90	93	94	94	95	95
OK	85	85	84	90	91	92	92
OR	93	95	94	94	94	95	95
PA	87	92	93	95	93	97	98

RI	88	93	95	99	102	105	107	
SC	102	106	103	105	104	105	103	
TN	98	100	99	99	97	100	97	
TX	96	99	97	98	98	100	100	
UT	101	102	98	101	98	102	102	
VT	102	104	102	103	102	105	104	
VA	104	105	106	106	104	107	106	
WA	95	100	97	100	100	102	98	
WV	81	84	84	84	80	78	79	
WI	103	105	102	103	102	104	103	
								Over-all
Average	**100.5**	**102.6**	**102.8**	**104.5**	**103.6**	**105.7**	**105.1**	**103.5**
Average factor by which % of all expected deaths are higher in locked states than in free states								1.1

* The CDC counts New York City data separately from the rest of New York State. This was considered in the average, as if New York City were a different state. The CDC also includes data from Washington, DC. Therefore, there are 6 states on the left, and 44 states plus two cities, NYC and DC, on the right.

We now see that not only comparing neighboring states, free vs locked, but now looking at the entire United States, there is a consistent pattern: Free states show not only fewer than expected deaths during each week than previous years at the same times, but also free states in Spring of 2020 had a distinct survival advantage, and significantly lower mortality than locked states, when each state is compared with its own previous record. The factor by which locked states' mortality change (as percent of expected) exceeded free states' mortality change (as percent of expected) was consistently positive and by a factor of 1.08 to 1.11.

Conclusion

Because the free states did not have increased deaths from their data in previous years, but their neighboring locked states did average increased deaths over the free states from their data in previous years, by a factor that stayed within the narrow range of 1.08 to 1.11 through the seven weeks including the end of, and the easing of lockdown in most states, we can therefore conclude with certainty that lockdown did not reduce deaths in the US.

In fact, free states had decreased deaths from their data in previous years, but locked states on average did not have decreased deaths from their data in previous years. Therefore, we can conclude with certainty that lockdown did not reduce deaths. How is this conclusion certain? Because if a popular hypothesis is that A caused B (lockdowns caused reduced deaths), but we then learn that B never happened, then we can confidently surmise that A definitely did not cause B. Causation is very hard to prove, but lack of causation is very easy to prove, particularly when the effect never happened. We can be certain that A did not cause B, if we see that B never happened at all. Lockdown did happen in most US states, including the states surrounding the free states, which I examined. However, deaths were not reduced in those locked states, neither in comparison to their own historical mortality data on average, nor in comparison to their free neighbors. Total deaths from all causes were not reduced in the locked states, as we see from the above data.

This paper examined CDC data to determine whether reduction in deaths happened in lockdown states. That did not happen; therefore, there is nothing, including lockdowns, that has caused it to happen.

The conclusion and its supporting data impact future assessments of whether lockdown was an optimal strategy of state governments. A failure of lockdowns to reduce deaths must in the future be considered when weighed against the considerable damage, including political, economic, humanitarian, social and psychological damage, caused directly by lockdowns. In fact, some of these harmful societal impacts have likely resulted in the deaths that we see from the data shown have been more prevalent in the locked states.

Society's response to the phenomenon of COVID-19 led to the loss of 30 million to 40 million jobs in the US alone.[348] The US unemployment rate rose to 14.7%. [349] Unemployment's adverse effects are known to reverberate through families and communities and business sectors, and must be considered in the future, if lockdown is ever proposed again. The consistently worse (by 8 to 11%) mortality results that I showed in locked states over free states likely reflect the life-threatening consequences of mass unemployment. In fact, many of the locked states are currently at risk of locking down again, even though the damage that those states have already incurred from lockdown is clear from this study.

Civil liberties concerns are also paramount to those who value those liberties perhaps as highly as their own lives, aware of wars throughout American history and world history that were fought in defense of or to establish the same. Those liberties were challenged, curtailed and violated to various degrees throughout the US, as a consequence of lockdowns. Therefore, lockdowns had historic and far-reaching social, political and economic effects, but they did not reduce deaths, and therefore cannot be justified now or in the future. The timeframe of this study is limited, however, and a more thorough assessment of lockdown impact on mortality would be obtained by a study of more weeks than the seven examined herein.

Lockdowns hurt minorities disproportionately

At least some of the states that had strictly enforced lockdowns in the late spring of 2020 also had severe mortality, especially for communities of color.

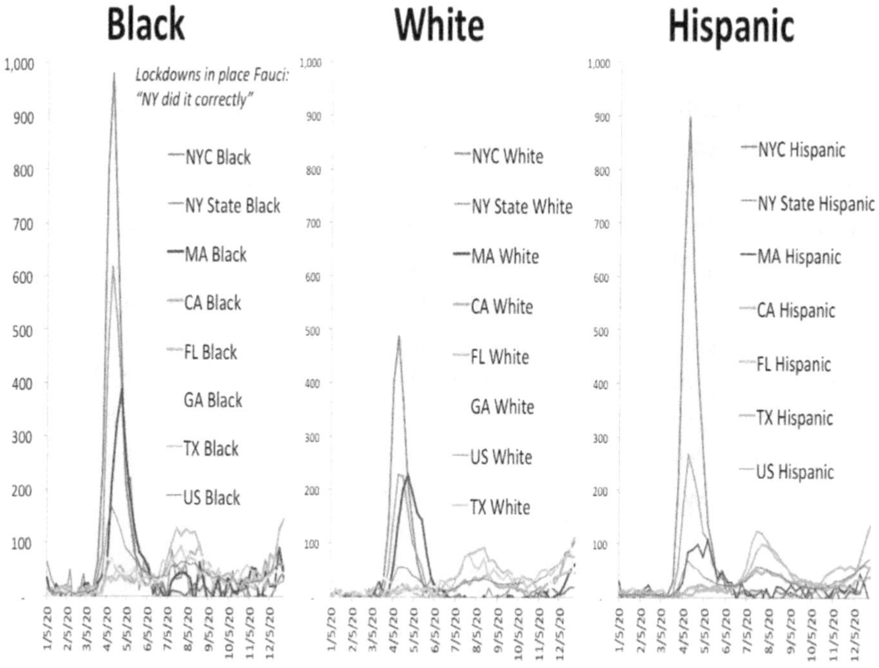

© Graphs by Emily Burns[350 351]

Lockdowns may have been associated with an enormous increase in deaths in minority populations, peaking in April 2020. Deaths attributed to COVID-19 also peaked sharply in April 2020, and disproportionate rates of deaths among minorities were alleged to be caused by COVID-19. However, if COVID-19 were the sole cause of the excess deaths, then states that had less stringent lockdowns might be expected to have had similar patterns in their mortality peaks.

These graphs do not conclusively prove that lockdowns have disproportionately harmed minority populations, but lockdowns in such strict areas as New York City, New York State and Massachusetts are seen in the above graphs to have not at all benefited people of color with regard to mortality. Unfortunately, because of the COVID-19 diagnosing and reporting flaws and miscalculations discussed in the first chapter of this book, the highly unlikely but thorough disappearance of seasonal influenza, and unlikely reductions in other diseases, it will likely never be known to what extent deaths attributed to COVID-19 were in fact due to other causes.[352] Therefore, it is possible that typical causes of deaths as well as lockdown-caused deaths were under-reported. These phenomena must be studied urgently, especially prior to any consideration of repeated lockdown, with consideration for not further harming vulnerable communities or the population at large.

We can also examine other parameters graphed against stringency of lockdowns. Burns' analysis continues in the following graphs:

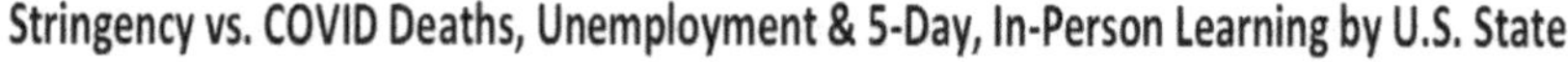

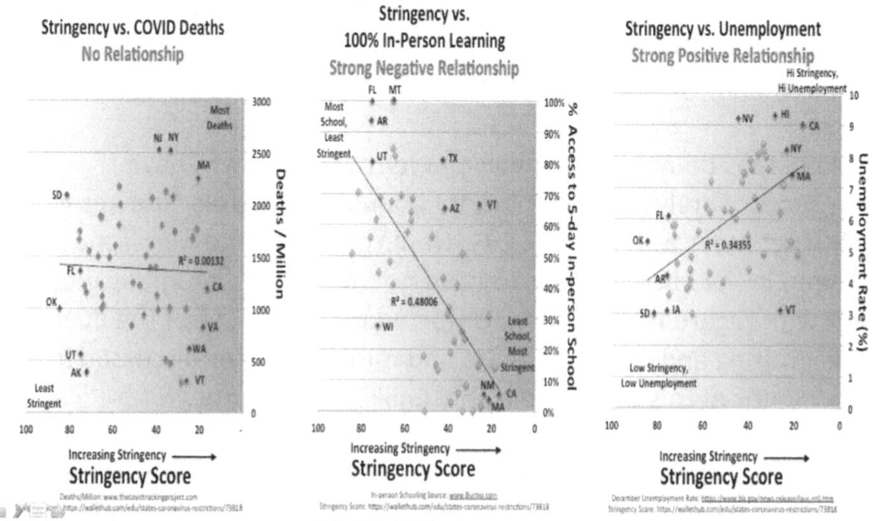

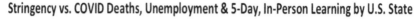

© Graphs by Emily Burns [353] [354] [355] [356]

Some of the data graphed are from US government websites. Not all data presented are peer-reviewed. However, there is enough of a concern raised by the strong inverse correlations between states that have had stringent lockdowns and such essential life needs as childhood education and employment. Vulnerable and minority communities as well as parents and children of all races are significantly impacted by the high unemployment rates and closed schools that still plague populations in the most severely restricted states.

Social Distancing

Throughout human history, quarantine of the ill has been a part of infectious diseases outbreak customs and protocol, formal and informal. Only in the most severe outbreaks was quarantine considered for the healthy. In the 14th century, at a time when the bubonic plague killed 25 million people in Europe, ships arriving to Venice were ordered to quarantine for 40 days.[357] Social distancing was an early 19th century concept that was discussed regarding tuberculosis patients. The arbitrary distance of six feet was suggested to avoid transmission.

More sinister applications of social distancing include 19th century British class elitism, as well as racism and racial segregation in the US of that time.[358] Social distancing in the 20th century was manifest in Jim Crow laws and practices, rooted in racial prejudice and racist hostility. Sociologist Robert Park defined social distance as "an attempt to reduce to something like measurable terms the grades and degrees of understanding and intimacy which characterize personal and social relations generally."[359]

The Bogardus Social Distance Scale, developed by American sociologist Emory Bogardus in 1924, was used to measure racial prejudice. Bogardus was known for his appreciation of ethnic and racial diversity, and worked for the All Nations Foundation and participated in the International Institute of Los Angeles, which assisted immigrants to adjust to society in the US. He wrote, "As a sociologist, I learned long ago that the human race is one, with similar problems and with a universal need for encouragement of many kinds."[360] He considered race divisions to be one of the US's major problems. The Bogardus Social Distance Scale consisted of four concentric circles in which close relations were in the smallest circle, followed by a larger circle of friends, a wider circle of acquaintances and the outside circle reserved for "enemies."

A later definition of social distance is the degree of intimacy and understanding that exists between individuals or social groups." Conversely, prejudice was defined as the "more or less instinctive and spontaneous disposition to maintain social distances" away from other groups.[361] Until 2020, social distance had been observed in spontaneous human activity. Since the spring of 2020, "social distancing" became an active practice, encouraged by government and media. To what extent would the deliberate act of creating distance place other people in successively farther groups on the Bogardus Scale? Did it make acquaintances of friends, or even enemies of acquaintances? Did it serve or create any divide-and-conquer political phenomena?

Returning to medicine and human health, attitudes toward sick people have made them the objects of empathy as well as avoidance, as it had long been practiced to isolate the sick at home and the very sick in hospitals. Never in recorded history had social distancing been taken to the extreme of Nazi Germany, where it was practiced in society-wide measures with uninfected people, and there had been no scientific studies nor historical experiences to support such a practice.[362] No scientific evidence had supported the value of distancing in a preventive way.[363] It was dismissed by the World Health Organization in 2006 as "ineffective and impractical."[364] Then after the appearance of the COVID-19 phenomenon, a new rule and a metric took hold throughout most of the world: People were instructed to stay six feet away from each other in 2020. Then in 2021, the new advice was three feet apart.

Whereas throughout human history, quarantine had almost exclusively involved those with signs and/or symptoms of infectious disease, in 2020 everyone was informed that they were "asymptomatic carriers." And everyone consequently was advised to socially distance from others. US government officials first explored the idea in 2005, after hearing of a 14-year old high school student's science fair project in which she built a model of people with fixed minimal distances among them.[365]

Did isolation of healthy people make any scientific sense? Former FDA Commissioner Scott Gottlieb MD said of the 6-foot distancing guideline, "This six-foot distancing requirement has probably been the single costliest mitigation tactic that we've employed in response to COVID . . . and it really wasn't based on clear science. . . . . We should have re-adjudicated this much earlier." And that it "might have been the single costliest measure" recommended by the US Centers for Disease Control and Prevention (CDC) and that "we don't know the exact basis for its initial view to stay 6 feet apart."[366] Indeed, there is no scientific basis for doing so, and no randomized controlled trials (RCTs) that show value of this practice. There is a meta-analysis funded by the World Health Organization of 172 observational studies regarding the practice,[367] but none of those studies is a RCT. Only seven of them were comparative for SARS-CoV-2, and none found any transmission from an asymptomatic person at any distance. Across all of the studies, a 10.2% lower risk was attributed to physical distancing of one meter or more, compared to closer than one meter. However, there was not a finding of transmission by an asymptomatic person to another, which is the basis of society-wide social distancing guidelines and the closing of schools, with the sacrifice of a year of education in the lives of children and youth.

An assumption that social distancing might have worked began because "cases" are no longer defined as they had been throughout history. Whereas a case of any disease was defined as a person with a set of signs and / symptoms of disease diagnosed by a physician, now it is quite different. The very sensitive PCR process of testing is a procedure that multiplies even a very small amount of genetic material up to a level beyond a threshold where it is "detected." Setting cycle thresholds at a high number, the "PCR test" becomes a self-fulfilling objective: more cases appear. The reported "cases" are specimens from individuals likely to contain nothing more than viral debris from prior infections with SARS-CoV-2 or other coronaviruses. Given that coronaviruses are approximately 30% of all cases of the common cold, it is not easy to find someone with that residue of a prior infection apparent on an overly sensitive "test."

Social distancing is only applicable to populations if it is first assumed that anybody may be infected with transmissible pathogens. In order to enact such a policy as social distancing, it must first be assumed that asymptomatic transmission is possible.

Nature published a study of the entire Wuhan population, involving 9,899,828 people. "There were no positive tests among 1,174 close contacts of asymptomatic cases."[368] A University of Florida meta-analysis of total 77,758 participants, found 0.7% new positive PCR tests in the presence of asymptomatic people of the same household with positive PCR tests, but did not exclude the possibility of infection acquired from outside the home.[369] One must also consider in each of the above-mentioned studies the highly dubious parameters for cycle thresholds of RT-PCR "tests" for SARS-CoV-2.

Immunologist Beda Stadler, former director of the Institute for Immunology at the University of Bern, discusses the widespread acceptance by western politicians and journalists of "asymptomatic transmission." He famously claimed that the notion of "asymptomatic transmission" of a virus was "the crowning of stupidity." [370] He explained that when someone is already immune, in the case of SARS 2, it was likely that a prior encounter with SARS 1, even at its peak 17 years earlier, or other past coronavirus encounter likely caused that outcome, and resulted in antibody presence. Such antibody presence and activity against new virus exposure doesn't mean the virus won't activate immune system cells, or won't bind cells before antibodies get to them, but neither is that a state of disease. Moreover, in new encounters with infectious pathogens, as T-cells search for any cells that may be incubating the virus throughout the body, such cytotoxic T-cell process continues until the last viral host cell is dead. The individual may remain asymptomatic as long as this process continues, and would not have nearly enough viral burden to share with another person.

Should the well submit to social distancing dictates? Epidemiologist Boris Borovoy explained, "If I don't have enough of a viral load to make myself sick, how could I possibly transmit enough viral load to make another person sick?"

PDMJ

Masks are neither effective nor safe: A summary of the science

Colleen Huber, NMD

First published as pre-print July 6, 2020
Peer review completed November 19, 2020

https://pdmj.org/papers/masks_are_neither_effective_nor_safe/index.html

Abstract

In 2020 there is a surge in use of facemasks in public places, including for extended periods of time, in the United States as well as in other countries. The public has been instructed by media and their governments that one's use of masks, even if not sick, may prevent others from being infected with SARS-CoV-2, the infectious agent of COVID-19.

A review of the peer-reviewed medical literature examines impacts of masks on human health, both immunological, as well as physiological. The purpose of this paper is to examine data regarding the effectiveness of facemasks, as well as safety data. The reason that both are examined in one paper is that for the general public as a whole, as well as for each individual, a risk-benefit analysis is necessary to guide decisions on if and when to wear a mask.

Are masks effective at preventing transmission of respiratory pathogens?

A 2020 meta-analysis found that face masks have no detectable effect against transmission of viral infections.[371] It found: "Compared to no masks, there was no reduction of influenza-like illness cases or influenza for masks in the general population, nor in healthcare workers."

Another 2020 meta-analysis, published by the US Centers for Disease Control (CDC), found that evidence from randomized controlled trials of face masks did not support a substantial effect on transmission of laboratory-confirmed influenza, either when worn by infected persons (source control) or by persons in the general community to reduce their susceptibility.[372]

Yet another 2020 analysis, found that masks had no effect specifically against Covid-19, although facemask use seemed linked to, in 3 of 31 studies, "very slightly reduced" odds of developing influenza-like illness.[373] The remainder of the 31 studies did not verify that finding.

A 2019 study of 2862 participants showed that both N95 respirators and surgical masks "resulted in no significant difference in the incidence of laboratory confirmed influenza."[374]

A 2016 meta-analysis found that both randomized controlled trials and observational studies of N95 respirators and surgical masks used by healthcare workers did not show benefit against transmission of acute respiratory infections. It was also found that acute respiratory infection transmission "may have occurred via contamination of provided respiratory protective equipment during storage and reuse of masks and respirators throughout the workday."[375]

A 2011 meta-analysis of 17 studies regarding masks and effect on transmission of influenza found that "none of the studies established a conclusive relationship between mask/respirator use and protection against influenza infection."[376] However, authors speculated that effectiveness of masks may be linked to early, consistent and correct usage.

Face mask use was likewise found to be not protective against the common cold, compared to controls without face masks among healthcare workers.[377]

Airflow around masks

Masks have been assumed to be effective in obstructing forward travel of viral particles. Considering those positioned next to or behind a mask wearer, there have been farther transmission of virus-laden fluid particles from masked individuals than from unmasked individuals, by means of "several leakage jets, including intense backward and downwards jets that may present major hazards," and a "potentially dangerous leakage jet of up to several meters."[378] All masks were thought to reduce forward airflow by 90% or more over wearing no mask. However, Schlieren imaging showed that both surgical masks and cloth masks had farther brow jets (upward airflow past eyebrows) than not wearing any mask at all, 182 mm and 203 mm respectively, vs none discernible with no mask. Backward airflow was found to be strong with all masks compared to not masking.

For both N95 and surgical masks, it was found that expelled particles from 0.03 to 1 micron were deflected around the edges of each mask, and that there was measurable penetration of particles through the filter of each mask.[379]

Penetration through masks

A study of 44 mask brands found mean 35.6% penetration (± 34.7%). Most medical masks had over 20% penetration, while "general masks and handkerchiefs had no protective function in terms of the aerosol filtration efficiency." The study found that "Medical masks, general masks, and handkerchiefs were found to provide little protection against respiratory aerosols."[380]

It may be helpful to remember that an aerosol is a colloidal suspension of liquid or solid particles in a gas. In respiration, the relevant aerosol is the suspension of bacterial or viral particles in inhaled or exhaled breath.

In another study, penetration of cloth masks by particles was almost 97% and medical masks 44%.[381]

N95 respirators

Honeywell is a manufacturer of N95 respirators. These are made with a 0.3 micron filter.[382] N95 respirators are so named, because 95% of particles having a diameter of 0.3 microns are filtered by the mask forward of the wearer, by use of an electrostatic mechanism. Coronaviruses are approximately 0.125 microns in diameter.

A meta-analysis found that N95 respirators did not provide superior protection to facemasks against viral infections or influenza-like infections.[383] Another study did find superior protection by N95 respirators when they were fit-tested compared to surgical masks.[384]

Another study found that 624 out of 714 people wearing N95 masks left visible gaps when putting on their own masks.[385]

Surgical masks

A 2010 study found that surgical masks offered no protection at all against influenza.[386] Another study found that surgical masks had about 85% penetration ratio of aerosolized inactivated influenza particles and about 90% of Staphylococcus aureus bacteria, although S aureus particles were about 6 times the diameter of influenza particles.[387]

Use of masks in surgery were found to slightly *increase* incidence of infection over not masking in a study of 3,088 surgeries.[388] The surgeons' masks were found to give no protective effect to the patients.

Other studies found no difference in wound infection rates with and without surgical mask use during surgery.[389] [390]

A 2015 study found that "there is a lack of substantial evidence to support claims that facemasks protect either patient or surgeon from infectious contamination."[391]

A 2020 study found that medical masks have a wide range of filtration efficiency, with most showing a 30% to 50% efficiency.[392]

Specifically, are surgical masks effective in stopping human transmission of coronaviruses? Both experimental and control groups, masked and unmasked respectively, were found to "not shed detectable virus in respiratory droplets or aerosols."[393] In that study, they "did not confirm the infectivity of coronavirus" as found in exhaled breath.

A study of aerosol penetration showed that two of the five surgical masks studied had 51% to 89% penetration of polydisperse aerosols.[394]

In another study, that observed subjects while coughing, "neither surgical nor cotton masks effectively filtered SARS-CoV-2 during coughs by infected patients." And more viral particles were found on the outside than on the inside of masks tested.[395]

Cloth masks

Cloth masks were found to have low efficiency for blocking particles of 0.3 microns and smaller. Aerosol penetration through a variety of cloth masks examined was found to be between 74 and 90%. The filtration efficiency of fabric materials was 3% to 33%[396]

Healthcare workers wearing cloth masks were found to have 13 times the risk of influenza-like illness than those wearing medical masks.[397]

This 1920 analysis of cloth mask use during the 1918 pandemic examines the failure of masks to impede or stop flu transmission at that time, and concluded that the number of layers of fabric required to prevent pathogen penetration would have required a suffocating number of layers, and could not be used for that reason, as well as the problem of leakage vents around the edges of cloth masks.[398]

A 2020 Duke University study found that a likely reason for the poor effect of cloth masks is that the mesh of the mask dispersed larger expired respiratory droplets "into a multitude of smaller droplets . . . which explains the apparent increase in droplet count relative to no mask in that case." It was also noted that those smaller particles are likely to stay airborne longer than larger droplets, which resulted in "counterproductive" use of these cloth masks.[399]

Masks against COVID-19

The New England Journal of Medicine editorial on the topic of mask use versus Covid-19 assesses the matter as follows:

> "We know that wearing a mask outside health care facilities offers little, if any, protection from infection. Public health authorities define a significant exposure to Covid-19 as face-to-face contact within 6 feet with a patient with symptomatic Covid-19 that is sustained for at least a few minutes (and some say more than 10 minutes or even 20 minutes). The chance of catching Covid-19 from a passing interaction in a public space is therefore minimal. In many cases, the desire for widespread masking is a reflexive reaction to anxiety over the pandemic."[400]

Are masks safe?

During walking or other exercise

Surgical mask wearers had significantly increased dyspnea after a 6-minute walk than non-mask wearers.[401]

Researchers are concerned about possible burden of facemasks during physical activity on pulmonary, circulatory and immune systems, due to oxygen reduction and air trapping reducing substantial carbon dioxide exchange. As a result of hypercapnia, there may be cardiac overload, renal overload, and a shift to metabolic acidosis.[402]

Risks of N95 respirators

Pregnant healthcare workers were found to have a loss in volume of oxygen consumption by 13.8% compared to controls when wearing N95 respirators. 17.7% less carbon dioxide was expired.[403] Patients with end-stage renal disease were studied during use of N95 respirators. Their partial pressure of oxygen (PaO2) decreased significantly compared to controls and increased respiratory adverse effects.[404] 19% of the patients developed various degrees of hypoxemia while wearing the masks.

Healthcare workers' N95 respirators were considered as personal bio-aerosol samplers, for collecting influenza virus.[405] And 25% of healthcare workers' facepiece respirators were found to contain influenza in an emergency department during the 2015 flu season.[406]

Risks of surgical masks

Healthcare workers' surgical masks were considered as "personal bio-aerosol samplers" and were found to collect and to harbor influenza virus.[407]

Various respiratory pathogens were found on the outer surface of used medical masks, which could result in self-contamination. The risk was found to be higher with longer duration of mask use.[408]

Surgical masks were also found to be a repository of bacterial contamination. The source of the bacteria was determined to be the body surface of the surgeons, rather than the operating room environment.[409] Given that surgeons are gowned from head to foot for surgery, this finding should be especially concerning for laypeople who wear masks. Without the protective garb of surgeons, laypeople generally have even more exposed body surface to serve as a source for bacteria to collect on their masks.

Risks of cloth masks

Healthcare workers wearing cloth masks had significantly higher rates of influenza-like illness after four weeks of continuous on-the-job use, when compared to controls.[410]

The increased rate of infection in mask-wearers may be due to a weakening of immune function during mask use. Surgeons have been found to have lower oxygen saturation after surgeries even as short as 30 minutes.[411] Low oxygen induces hypoxia-inducible factor 1 alpha (HIF-1). This in turn down-regulates CD4+ T-cells.[412] CD4+ T-cells, in turn, are necessary for viral immunity.[413]

Weighing risk versus benefit of mask use

In 2020 the United States is seeing an unprecedented surge of mask use by the public. Homemade and store-bought cloth masks and surgical masks or N95 masks are being used by the public especially when entering stores and other publicly accessible buildings. Sometimes bandanas or scarves are used. The use of face masks, whether cloth, surgical or N95, creates a poor obstacle to aerosolized pathogens as we can see from the meta-analyses and other studies in this paper, allowing both transmission of aerosolized pathogens to others in various directions, as well as self-contamination. Forward projection of exhaled material may be partly replaced by lateral, backward, downward and upward projection, and to greater distances, with longer time airborne, from a masked person than from an unmasked person.

It must also be considered that masks impede the necessary volume of air intake required for adequate oxygen / carbon dioxide exchange, which results in observed physiological effects that may be undesirable. Even 6-minute walks, let alone more strenuous activity, resulted in dyspnea. The volume of unobstructed oxygen in a typical breath is about 100 ml, used for normal physiological processes. 100 ml O2 greatly exceeds the volume of a pathogen required for transmission.

The foregoing data show that masks serve more as instruments of obstruction of normal breathing, rather than as effective barriers to pathogens. Therefore, masks should not be used by the general public, either by adults or children, and their limitations as prophylaxis against pathogens should also be considered in medical settings. The clinical studies and meta-analyses that are referenced, cited and linked herein are presented in order to provide the best opportunity for informed decision-making, and for individuals to consider and compare the risks versus benefits of mask use.

PDMJ

Masks, false safety and real dangers, Part 1:

Friable mask particulate and lung vulnerability

September 13, 2020.
Completed peer-review and revised, September 24, 2020

Boris Borovoy,[iv] Colleen Huber,[v] Q Makeeta[vi]

https://pdmj.org/papers/masks_false_safety_and_real_dangers_part1/

[iv] Boris A Borovoy, MPH has a Master in Public Health from Moscow Medical Academy.

[v] Colleen Huber, NMD is a Naturopathic Medical Doctor and Naturopathic Oncologist (FNORI), writing on topics of masks, COVID-19, cancer and nutrition.

[vi] Q Makeeta, DC is a Doctor of Chiropractic.

Abstract

There is no biological history of mass masking until the current era. It is important to consider possible outcomes of this society-wide experiment. The consequences to the health of individuals is as yet unknown.

Masked individuals have measurably higher inspiratory flow than non-masked individuals. This study is of new masks removed from manufacturer packaging, as well as a laundered cloth mask, examined microscopically. Loose particulate was seen on each type of mask. Also, tight and loose fibers were seen on each type of mask. If every foreign particle and every fiber in every facemask is always secure and not detachable by airflow, then there should be no risk of inhalation of such particles and fibers. However, if even a small portion of mask fibers is detachable by inspiratory airflow, or if there is debris in mask manufacture or packaging or handling, then there is the possibility of not only entry of foreign material to the airways, but also entry to deep lung tissue, and potential pathological consequences of foreign bodies in the lungs.

Introduction

The nose and mouth are the gateways to the lungs for land vertebrates. There is no known history of a species that has begun to voluntarily or involuntarily obstruct, partially obstruct or filter the orifices to their airways and lungs. We have no biological history of such a species or how they would have adapted to or possibly survived such a novel practice.

However, recently, in mid-2020, throughout the world, in some countries far more than others, human self-masking has become commonplace, whether due to insistence by governments, requirement of employers, educational institutions and business-owners, or social pressures in one's immediate social circles. The proximal reason behind these reasons is abundant fear and desire for protection from COVID-19 throughout the world in 2020. People have been either coerced or otherwise pressured to wear "face coverings," allegedly for the purpose of "slowing the spread of COVID-19." The general public's response is to use disposable surgical masks, and a wide variety of cloth masks and other cloth face coverings. In the western hemisphere at least these facemasks had not been worn outside of certain hospital facilities, not outside of surgical settings and intensive care units of hospitals.

Prior research has overwhelmingly shown that there is no significant evidence of benefits of masks, particularly regarding transmission of viral infections, and that there are well-established risks. Evidence from peer-reviewed clinical studies and meta-analyses on problems concerning the effectiveness and safety of masks are summarized in this article.[414]

Optimal oxygen intake in humans has been calculated in the absence of any obstruction to the airways. The US Occupational Safety and Health Administration (OSHA) has determined that the optimal range of oxygen in the air for humans is between 19.5 and 23.5%. In previous times, before the COVID-19 era, OSHA required that any human-occupied airspace where oxygen measured less than 19.5% to be labelled as "not safe for workers."[415] The percentage of oxygen inside a masked airspace generally measures 17.4% within several seconds of wearing. It has been observed that maximal voluntary ventilation and maximal inspiratory pressure increase during lower availability of oxygen at ascent in altitude, [416] as well as for those who live at high altitude.[417] Because oxygen is so essential to life, and in adequate amounts, humans and animals have developed the ability to sense changes in oxygen concentration, and to adapt to such challenges quickly. The medulla oblongata and carotid bodies are sensitive to such changes. Both lower ambient oxygen and increased ambient carbon dioxide stimulates ventilation, as the body quickly and steadfastly attempts to acquire more oxygen.[418] As a compensatory mechanism, inspiratory flow is measurably higher in mask-wearers than in controls.[419]

The question then arises: If inspiratory flow is increased over normal while wearing a mask, is every fiber attached to one's facemask secure enough not to be inhaled into the lungs of the mask-wearer? Is it good enough for a majority of these fibers to be secure? Or must every part of every mask fiber of every mask be secure at all times?

Materials Used in Masks

Inhaled cotton fibers have been shown to cause subpleural ground glass opacities at the surface of the visceral pleura, as well as centrilobular and peribronchovascular interstitial thickening, as well as fibrous thickening of peribronchiolar interstitium. It was found by spectral analysis by infrared spectrophotometry that the foreign bodies in the lungs had an identical pattern to that of cellulose, which must have come from the inhaled cotton fibers.[420] Cotton and even silk may contribute to COPD in textile workers. Byssinosis is a pulmonary syndrome related to textile work. When textile workers were exposed to organic dusts from textiles in the workplace, both reversible and irreversible pulmonary conditions, such as asthma and COPD developed.[421] It should be remembered that unmasked textile workers would not have such high inspiratory flow as masked individuals.

Therefore, there is even more need that the fibers, debris and other particulate attached to cloth masks would stay entirely intact; every fiber, and every part of every fiber, and throughout every breath, at all times, even down to the size of nanometers.

Disposable surgical face masks are made of synthetic fibers, including polymers such as polypropylene, polyurethane, polyacrylonitrile, polystyrene, polycarbonate, polyethylene or polyester. There is an inner layer of soft fibers and a middle layer, which is a melt-blown filter, as well as a water-resistant outer layer of nonwoven fibers.[422] This study shows FT-IR spectra of the degrading fibers of disposable masks. It found that disposable face masks "could be emerging as a new source of microplastic fibers, as they can degrade/fragment or break down into smaller size/pieces . . . . [423]

Research on synthetic fibers has shown a correlation between the inhalation of synthetic fibers and various bronchopulmonary diseases, such as asthma, alveolitis, chronic bronchitis, bronchiectasis, fibrosis, spontaneous pneumothorax and chronic pneumonia. Cellular proliferation made up of histiocytes and fibroblasts were found in the lungs of those exposed to synthetic fibers in ambient air. Focal lesions in the lungs showed granulomas and collagen fibers containing both fine dust and long fibers. Some of the lung illnesses from this exposure could be reversed, while others had already proceeded to pulmonary fibrosis.[424]

Bioburden of masks has also been established. This study found bioburden on each type of mask studied, even after first use in a surgical environment. Speaking while wearing masks resulted in a significantly higher bioburden cultured from the face side of a mask.[425]

Possible Risk of Pulmonary Fibrosis

Pulmonary fibrosis is among the worst diseases that can be suffered or witnessed. It kills exceedingly slowly, by ever-thickening matrix formation, a kind of scar tissue, obstructing the alveoli and reducing their air exchange. The illness worsens slowly over time, and suffocates the victim very gradually. Nothing is available to the sufferer from conventional medicine. Neither medication nor radiation can undo the damage of the fibrous matrix laid down in the lungs' tissue. Similarly, surgery is not available to eliminate the insidious, suffocating mesh that painstakingly takes the life of the unfortunate patient. Neither is any known cure available in the realm of natural or alternative medicine. Neither nutrient, herb, nor any other known treatment can even reduce the fibrogenesis, let alone eliminate it. The 5-year survival rate is only 20%.[426] The only remedy against this scourge is diligent prevention of small and microscopic inhaled foreign bodies.

Inhaled particles, particularly nanoparticles, can begin the process of pulmonary fibrosis by forming free radicals such as superoxide anions. The resulting oxidative stress promotes inflammatory responses and surface reactivity.[427] The pathogenesis of idiopathic pulmonary fibrosis begins when Type 2 alveoli are injured and epithelia is not fully healed. Interstitial fibroblasts differentiate into myofibroblasts, which gather in fibrotic foci and form fibers with contractile properties.[428] This is followed by synthesis and deposit of extracellular matrix, which seems to be key in suffocating the air exchange of alveoli.

Particles of nanometer to micrometer size have been implicated as causative agents in pulmonary fibrosis.[429] Airborne inhaled nano-size particles are especially dangerous for the lungs, but are small enough to undergo transcytosis across epithelial and endothelial cells to enter blood and lymph, reaching the cardiovascular system, spleen, bone marrow, and have been observed to travel along axons and dendrites of the central nervous system and ganglia, a phenomenon that has been known for decades.[430]

Inhaled particles of 20 nm have deposited, more than other sizes of nano-particles, in the alveolar region, during nose-breathing of a person at rest.[431]

Methods

We examined microscopically the concave face side of a variety of new masks, taken directly out of their packaging from the manufacturer, not yet worn. However, the cloth mask below was worn for one day, and then laundered, and never worn again.

The following are the types of masks and the macroscopic view of the face side of each:

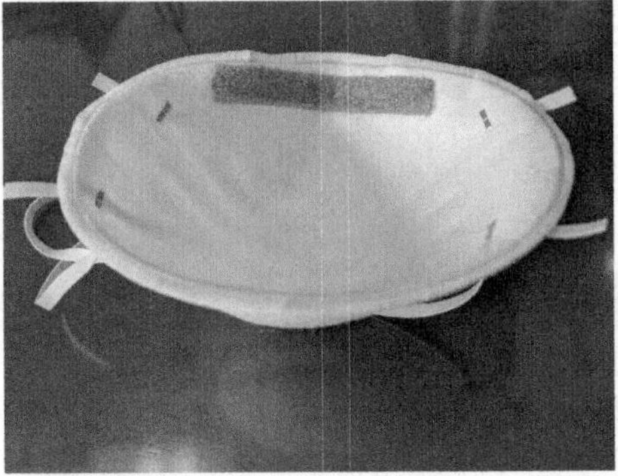

Cup mask

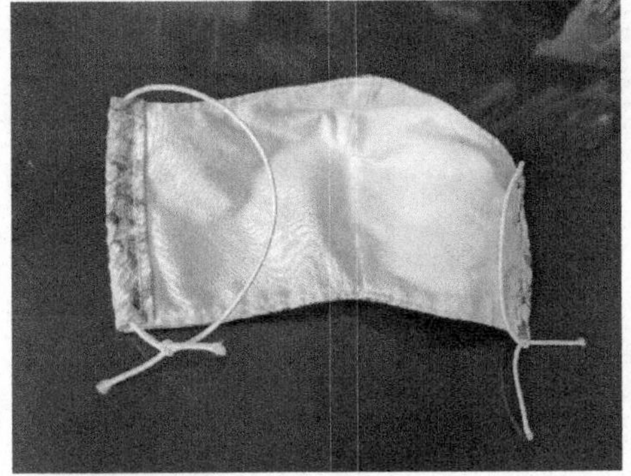

Cloth mask

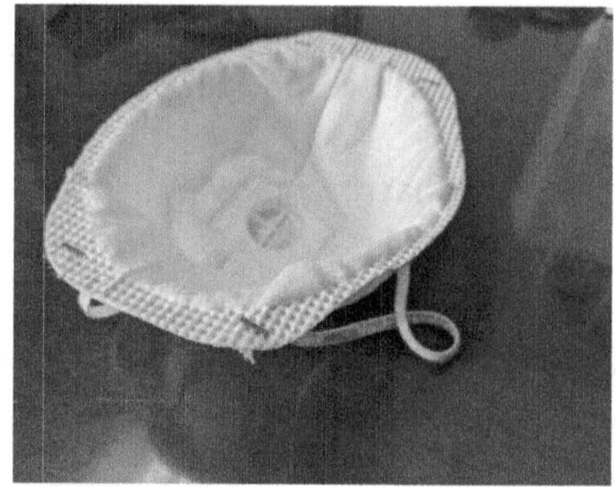

N-95 mask #1

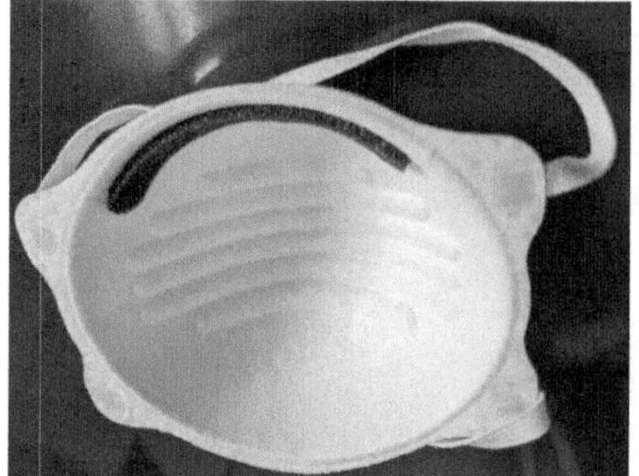

N-95 mask #2

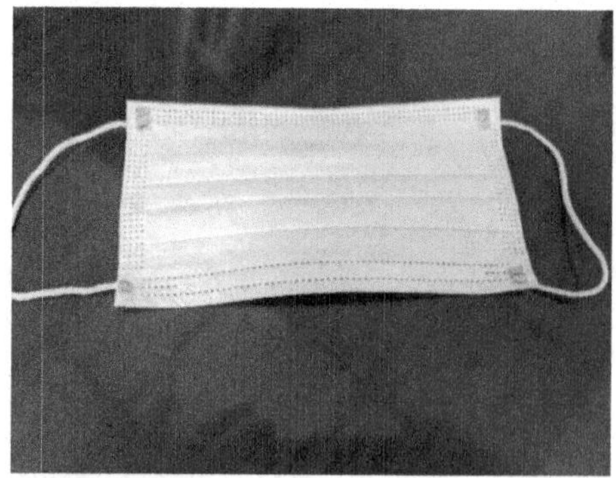

Surgical mask

The following photos were taken of the same masks at 40x to 100x magnification.

Higher resolution photos from other sources are in Appendix A.

Cup mask particulate and soiled appearing fibers

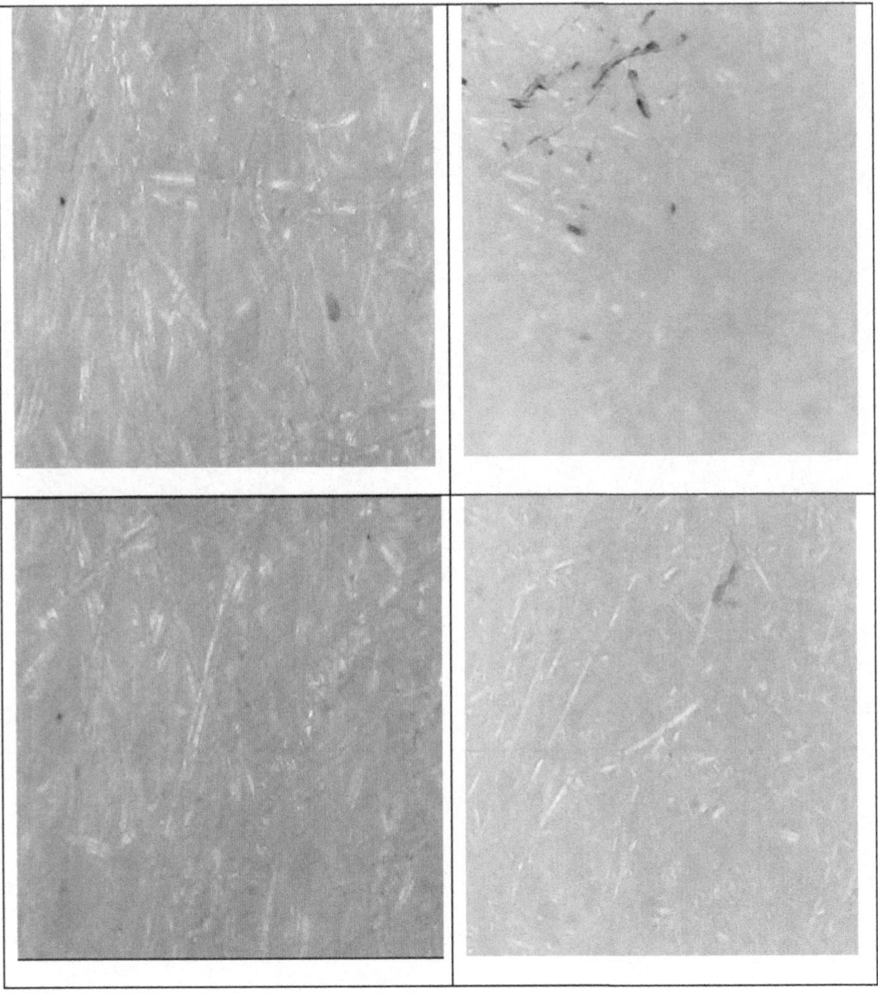

Cloth mask particulate and loosened fibers after one day use and laundering once

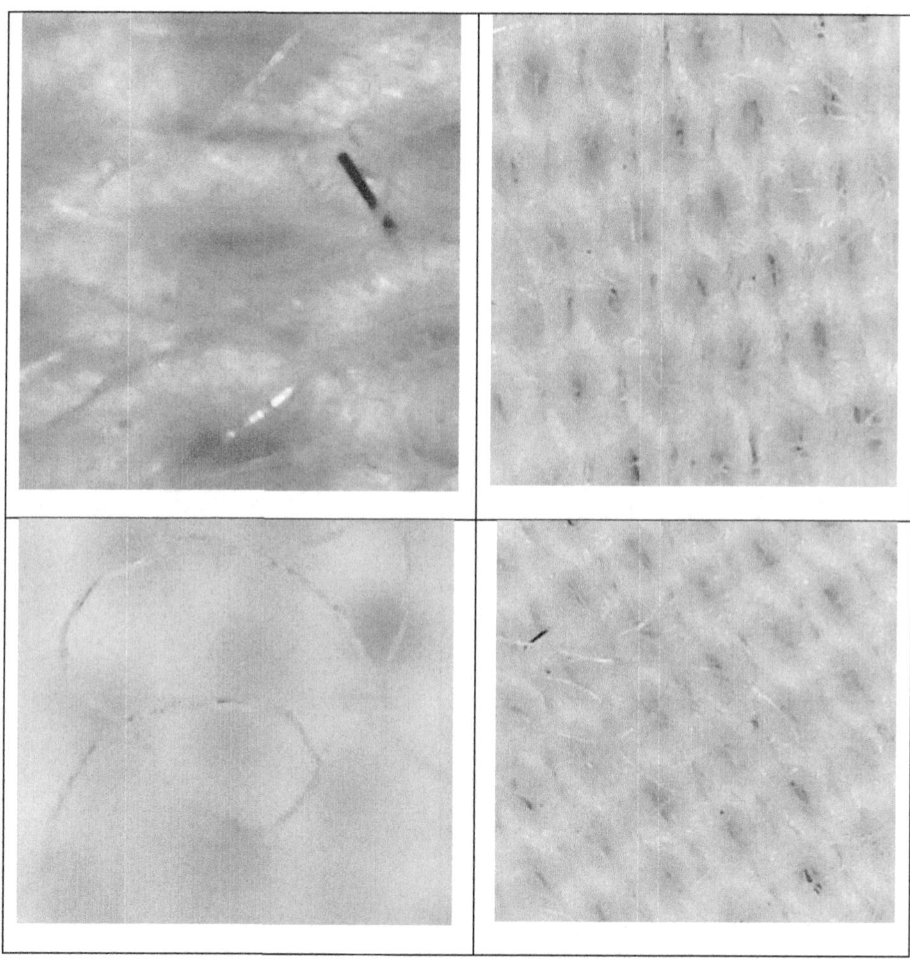

Surgical mask soiled appearance and particulate

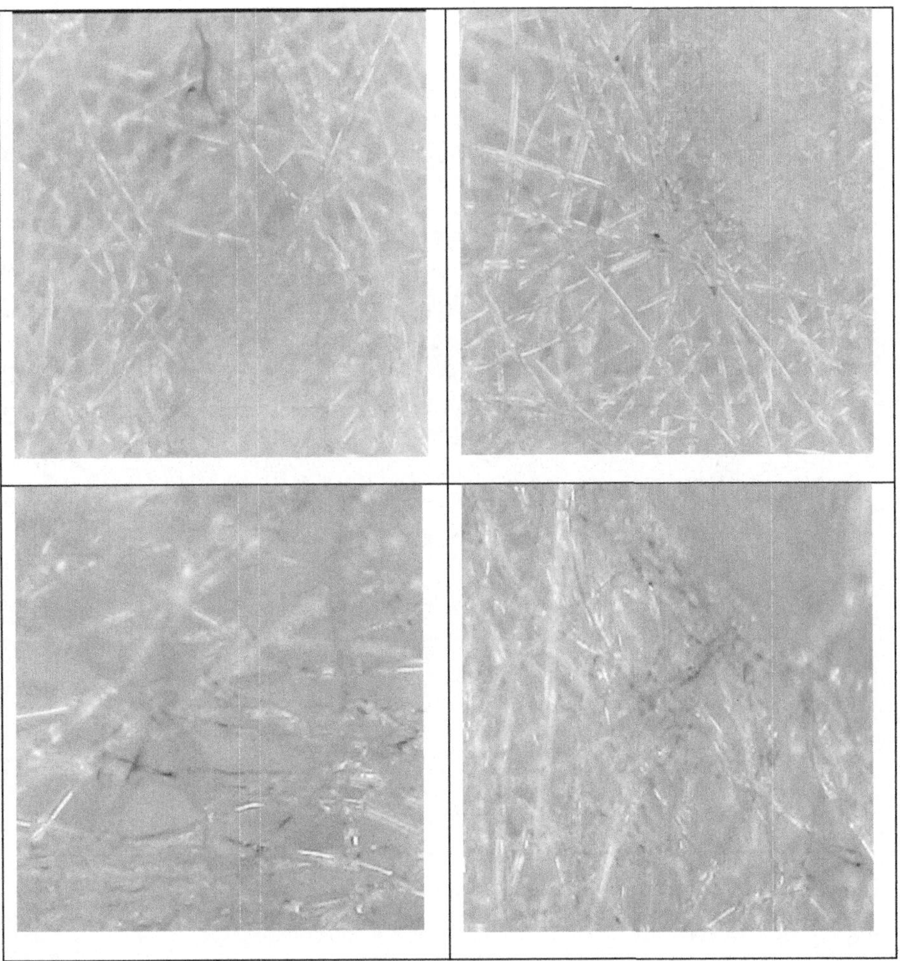

N-95 #1 particulate and soiled appearing fibers

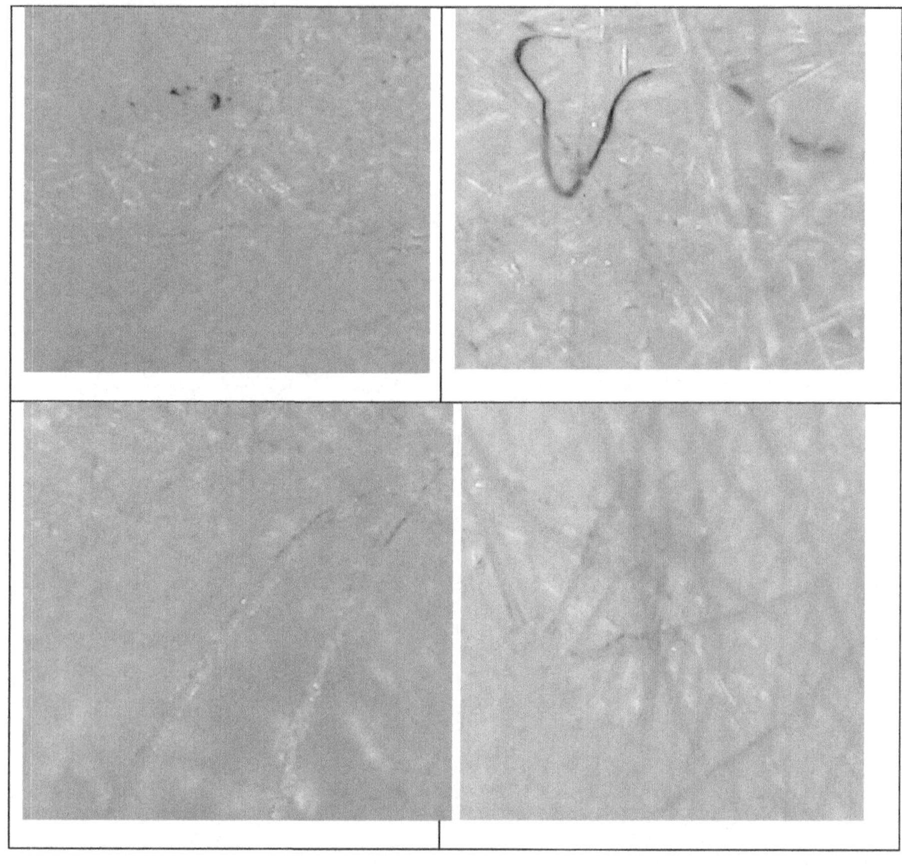

N-95 #2 particulate

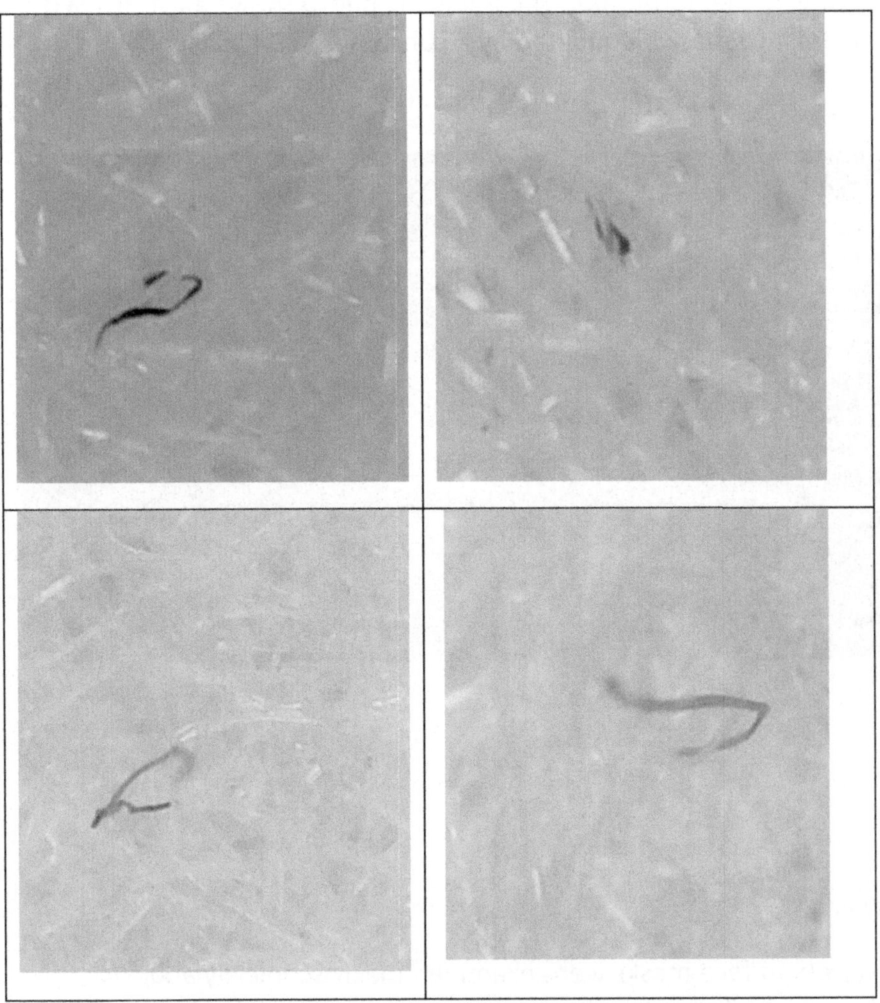

On the other hand, when masks are used, particulate and fibers may become further loosened. The following photo shows a lightly used hospital face mask illuminated by a consumer LED flashlight.

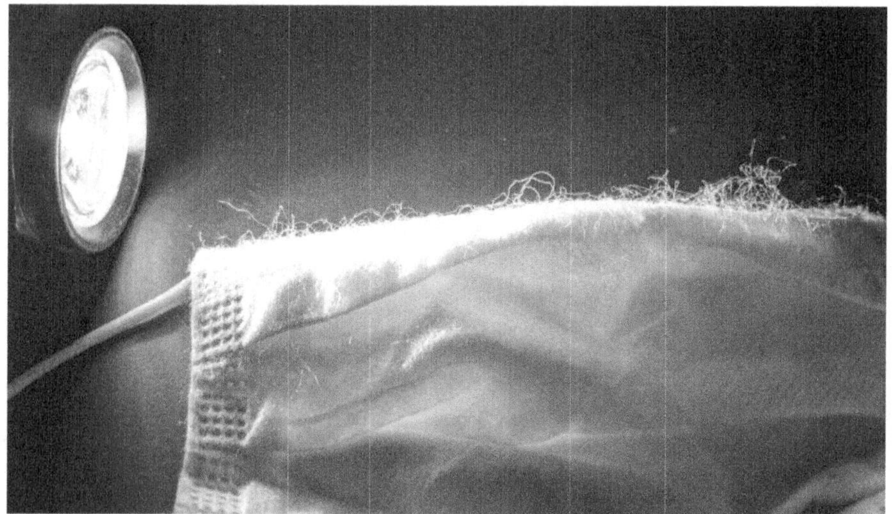

Results

A variety of face masks were examined macroscopically and microscopically. Each type of new, just unpackaged mask showed particulate matter and/or unidentified fibers. The first N-95 showed the fewest loose particles. All of the masks showed partially loose fibers in nearly every visual field. The cloth mask had been used previously but was laundered and then not used again. This also showed loose fibers dangling from the woven fabric of the mask, as well as particulate debris. The cloth mask had more loose fibers than the others, typically 4 or 5 partially loose or dangling fibers that were compressible toward the weave in each visual field.

The unclean appearance surrounding the oval shapes of the surgical mask may be due to an artifact of the thermal processing of mask textile. This may be some drops of melted polyethylene or other polymer plastic.

Conclusion

Surgical personnel are trained to never touch any part of a mask, except the loops and the nose bridge. Otherwise, the mask is considered useless and is to be replaced. Surgical personnel are strictly trained not to touch their masks otherwise. However, the general public may be seen touching various parts of their masks. Even the masks just removed from manufacturer packaging have been shown in the above photos to contain particulate and fiber that would not be optimal to inhale.

Both cotton and polymer clothing have been well-tolerated without pathology when covering any other part of the body, except over the only entry points/gateway to the respiratory system. Inhalation risks, such as the constant ventilation of the respiratory process, increased by the greater effort to attempt to fulfill bodily oxygen needs, with mostly and closely covered orifices are of great concern for those who would want to protect pulmonary health, without inhalation of unwanted particulate. When partial airway obstruction, i.e. masking, is added, deeper and more forceful breathing occurs. When this phenomenon is combined with the particles found herein on microscopic examination of the face side of newly unpackaged, never worn masks, there can arise the risk of a dangerous level of foreign material entering lung tissue. Furthermore, worn masks can only either lose these particles to lodge in the lungs of the wearer, or they would accumulate during use, to the burden (both biological and debris) of non-mask material carried on the inside of the mask.

Further concerns of macrophage response and other immune and inflammatory and fibroblast response to such inhaled particles specifically from facemasks should be the subject of more research.

If widespread masking continues, then the potential for inhaling mask fibers and environmental and biological debris continues on a daily basis for hundreds of millions of people. This should be alarming for physicians and epidemiologists knowledgeable in occupational hazards.

Appendix A

The following are higher resolution microscopic photos of masks, with links to the sources of the photos.

Disposable surgical masks, with scanning electron microscope views.

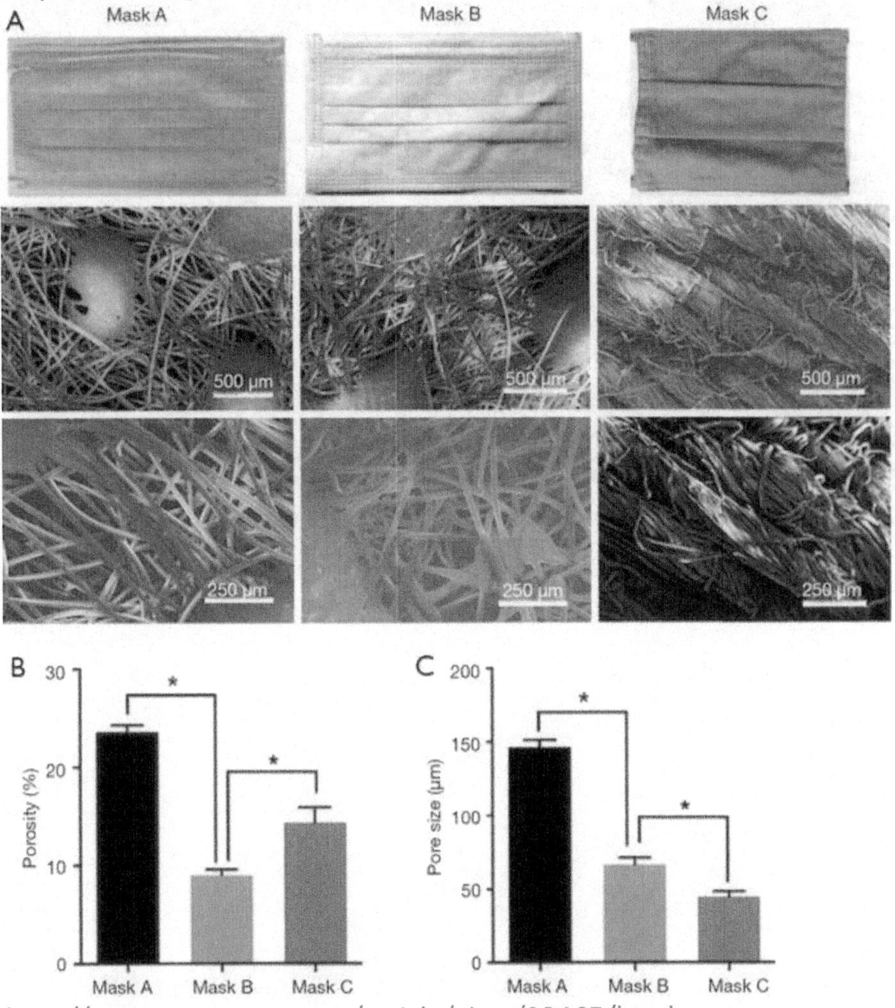

http://atm.amegroups.com/article/view/32465/html
http://cdn.amegroups.cn/journals/amepc/files/journals/16/articles/32465/public/32465-PB4-7346-R1.png

Cotton cloth photo at 40x magnification

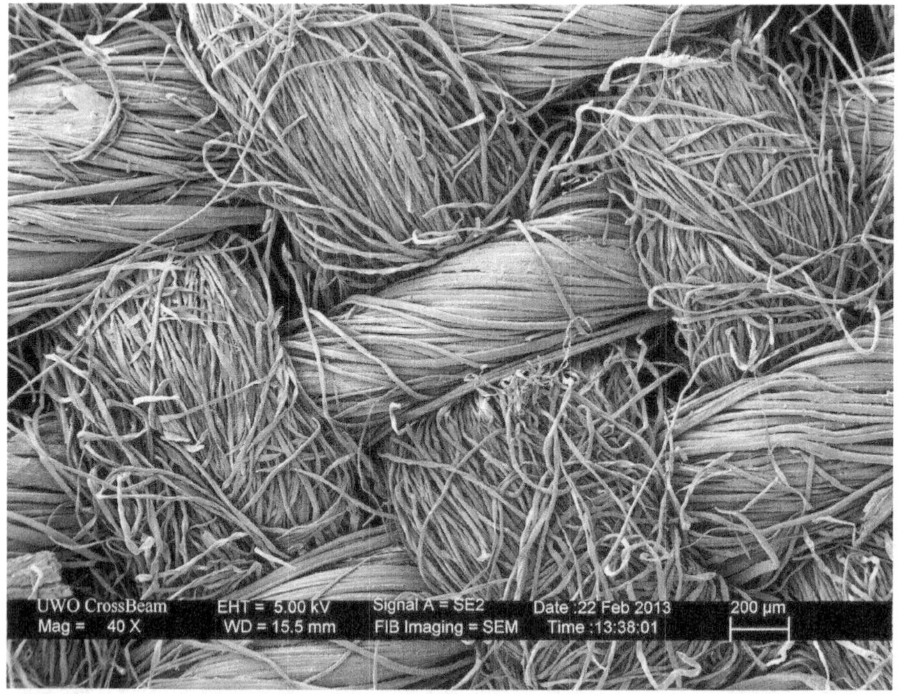

https://i.pinimg.com/originals/8e/cf/29/8ecf29ee6e2062ed0d92313042e58dd3.jpg

N-95 Respirator, at 20 micron resolution, scanning electron microscope

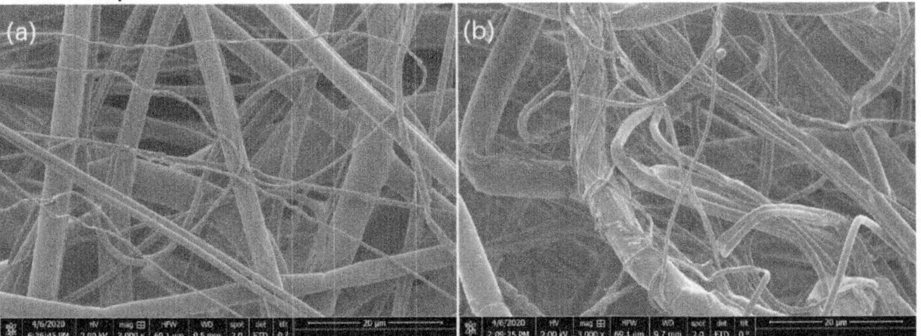

https://groups.oist.jp/sites/default/files/imce/u92/fmask/SEM200mu.png

PDMJ

Masks, false safety and real dangers, Part 2: Microbial challenges from masks

October 9, 2020.
Completed peer-review and revised, October 15, 2020

Boris Borovoy,[vii] Colleen Huber,[viii] Maria Crisler[ix]

https://pdmj.org/papers/masks_false_safety_and_real_dangers_part2/

Abstract

Face masks have come into common use in many countries since mid-2020, for all age groups. Some aspect of this may be voluntary, but certainly much of this use is either accompanied by force, threats, subtle coercion, or a continuum of subtle to fierce societal pressures on the individual to conform to mask-wearing. From widespread fear of COVID-19, associated with the virus named SARS-CoV2, mask-wearing is recently assumed by many to be a prudent measure against

---

[vii] Boris A Borovoy, MPH has a Master in Public Health from Moscow Medical Academy.

[viii] Colleen Huber, NMD is a Naturopathic Medical Doctor and Naturopathic Oncologist (FNORI), writing on topics of masks, COVID-19, cancer and nutrition.

[ix] Maria Crisler is a microbiologist.

contagion. In this paper, the second in our series, we continue our examination of the potential hazards of masks, in which we now turn attention to microbial contamination from masks and mask use, changes in oral and nasal microbiota, and potential risks to the lungs and other organ systems from microbial factors. Because widespread masking is a very new society-wide experiment, the impact of this experiment, the obstruction of airways from free breathing and a typical air exchange interplay with oral microbiota is not yet known. Furthermore, the effects of such changes in the lungs and beyond are not yet known. This paper will explore some considerations of these changes, by examining mask effectiveness against transmission, historical evidence of epidemiology from the 1918-1919 pandemic, microbial contamination, respiratory disease and the role of oral bacteria in systemic disease; and infections involving fungi, yeast, and molds. Compiling statistical and scientific evidence from these subjects alone should help equip any individual with adequate information on risks and benefits when choosing whether to wear a mask.

Are masks effective in preventing transmission of infection and are there unintended consequences when wearing them?

Face masks have been adopted by the public of several countries in 2020, with astonishing speed. Conflicting instructions from public health authorities left individual citizens unsure of whether to wear a mask, such that relying on gathered commentary from media and acquaintances in order to make such a decision has become standard. When an individual's preferences are not well formed, merely observing another person makes the option chosen by the other person a social default that is more likely to be chosen by the observer also.[432]

Concerns regarding use of masks among the public have been voiced by many medical professionals. Over 2,000 Belgian medical professionals, including hundreds of medical doctors, have urged prevention of COVID-19 by means of strengthening natural immunity.

Their recommendations, among other measures, include specifically to exercise in fresh air *without a mask.*[433] A number of reasons for this concern have been raised. In this paper, we will examine specifically microbial concerns with regard to mask-wearing.

Masks have been shown through overwhelming clinical evidence to have no effect against transmission of viral pathogens.[434] Penetration of cloth masks by viral particles was almost 97% and of surgical masks was 44%.[435] Even bacteria, approximately ten times the volume of coronaviruses, have been poorly impeded by both cloth masks and disposable surgical masks. Face masks became almost ineffective after two hours of use, and after 150 minutes of use, more bacteria was emitted through the disposable mask than from the same subject unmasked.[436] One must wonder, if new masks worn by healthcare workers, that are soiled by wear during a work shift, transmit more bacteria to patients than from an unmasked healthcare worker, then what is happening to the lungs of the mask-wearer?

Use of personal protective equipment (PPE) has long been debated for healthcare workers regarding their interactions with patients who are carrying highly pathogenic organisms, and this study found about half of even trained healthcare workers in clinical settings make at least one protocol deviation in donning and doffing PPE.[437] Certainly the general public without such training is likely to have a higher rate of similar or more egregious errors in PPE protocol. Masks have been determined to be unnecessary even in surgical settings, and of no benefit in preventing infections.[438] In fact, "The rate of wound infections [while unmasked] was less than half what it was when everyone wore masks." Oral microbial flora dispersed by unmasked healthcare workers standing one meter from the workspace failed to contaminate exposed plates on that surface.[439]

Let us also examine the entire surface area of the masked person when considering that person's potential for transmitting pathogens. Facemasks generally only cover the lower half of the face, which we know from studying burn victims is less than 2% of the entire body surface area.[440] We know that numbers of airborne bacteria expelled from the upper airway are insignificantly small compared with the volume of bacteria shed from the skin.[441] The bacteria shed from the skin of mask wearers was found to create more contamination than from non-mask wearers, presumably due to shifting, wiggling and increased rubbing and exfoliation.[442] [443]

The challenge to the masked person is that the lungs normally expel bacteria with freely exhaled breath, a necessary exhaust system not previously challenged throughout human or even vertebrate history with deliberate obstruction. In this paper we also explore both the effect of masks on microbial transmission as well as the risks and demonstrated problems of re-directed and re-inhaled bacteria and other microbes into the airways.

Are masks effective in preventing transmission of COVID-19 in particular?

COVID-19 is a remarkably low transmissibility disease. This paper shows patterns of transmission to close contacts from those who tested positive for SARS CoV2 in New South Wales high schools and primary schools. From 18 initial positive tests, only 2 out of 863 close contacts tested positive as a secondary case.[444]

In July 2020, the Council of Foreign Relations conducted a survey of 25 countries, with the following question to their citizens:

"Have you always worn a face mask outside the home in the last seven days?" The "Yes" responses ranged from 1% in Finland and Denmark, to 93% in Singapore.[445]
We then examined each of the same 25 countries for prevalence of mask use versus Covid-19 deaths per 1 million population. This data was gathered from Worldometers statistics.[446] That data is shown in Table 1, also represented in Graph 1.

Table 1

	% mask use over Jul 6-12, 2020 from CFR survey	Covid deaths per 1M pop, at 10/7/2020 from Worldometers
Singapore	93	5
Philippines	92	54
Brazil	90	694
UAE	89	44
India	88	76
Spain	87	696
Mexico	86	637
Hong Kong	85	14
Thailand	82	0.8
Indonesia	80	42
Italy	79	597
Saudi Arabia	79	142
Malaysia	76	4
Vietnam	68	0.4
China	67	3
United States	65	653
Germany	63	115
Taiwan	59	0.3
France	52	497
United Kingdom	22	625
Australia	12	35
Norway	3	51
Sweden	3	582
Denmark	1	114
Finland	1	62

Graph 1

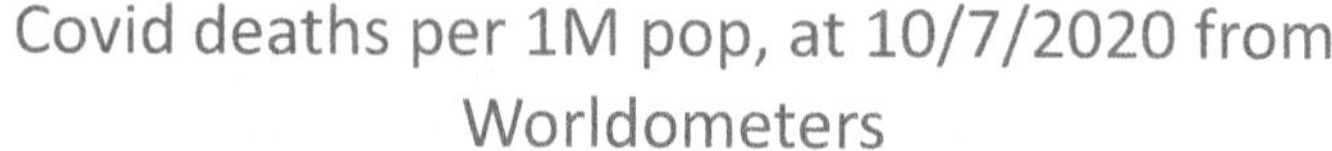

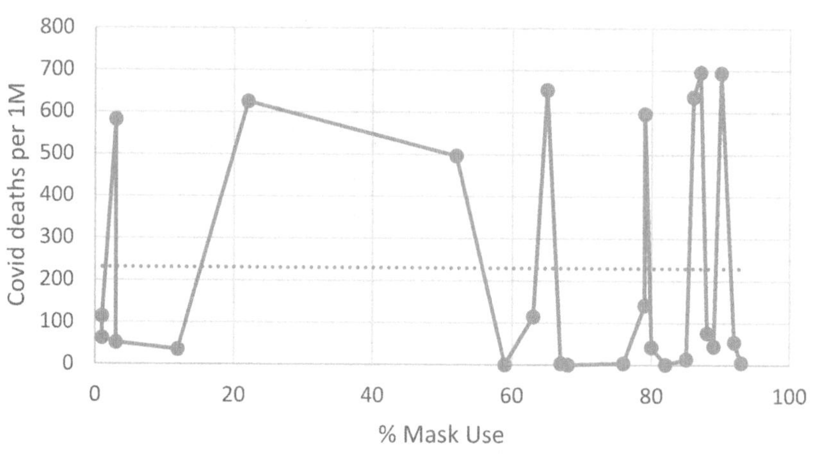

As we see from the above data, there was no significant correlation with mask use and either increase or reduction of deaths from COVID-19; thus masking could not have caused a significant reduction in deaths. In fact, two of the countries with the highest COVID-19 deaths also had high rates of mask use: Spain at 87% mask use and Brazil at 90% mask use. Again, masking could not have caused a significant reduction in deaths.

Another table presented from Worldometers data also demonstrates the rate of positive COVID-19 PCR tests per one million population in the same 25 countries surveyed. This data is reported in Table 2 and Graph 2.

Table 2

	% mask use over Jul 6-12, 2020 from CFR survey	Total + PCR tests per 1M pop, at 10/7/2020 from Worldometers
Singapore	93	9866
Philippines	92	2998
Brazil	90	23378
UAE	89	10264
India	88	4938
Spain	87	18654
Mexico	86	6146
Hong Kong	85	385
Thailand	82	52
Indonesia	80	1151
Italy	79	5525
Saudi Arabia	79	9661
Malaysia	76	431
Vietnam	68	11
China	67	59
United States	65	23385
Germany	63	3708
Taiwan	59	22
France	52	10006
United Kingdom	22	8006
Australia	12	1063
Norway	3	2742
Sweden	3	9557
Denmark	1	5297
Finland	1	1993

Graph 2

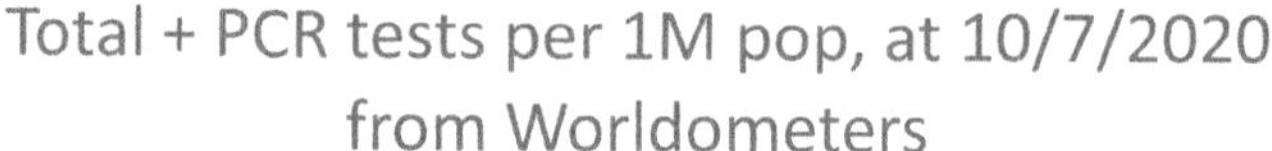
Total + PCR tests per 1M pop, at 10/7/2020
from Worldometers

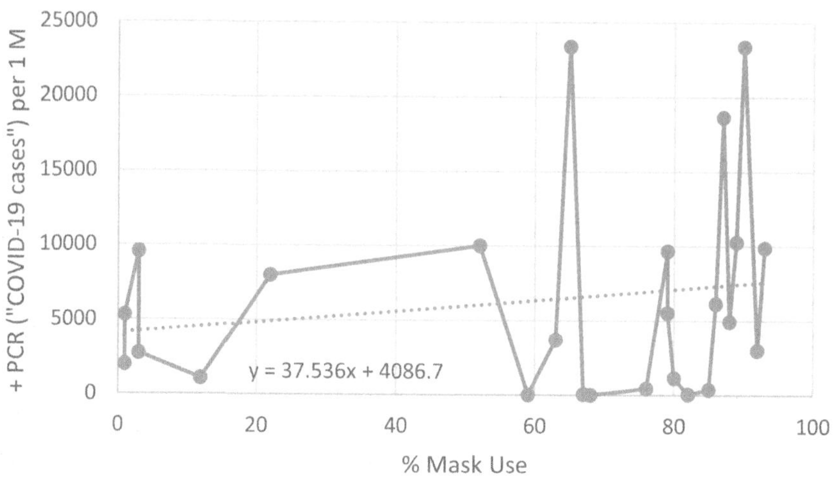

Contrary to data in table 1, we do see a significant trend in table 2. Curve-fitting a trend line, we see a positive slope for this line of 37.536. That is, for every increased percentage point of mask use in a country, there were an average of 37.536 additional positive PCR tests per one million population. This shows that masking has not accomplished the advertised function of reducing the number of positive PCR tests, but rather seems to be correlated with an increased number of positive PCR tests for COVID-19.

The historical role of bacteria in a viral pandemic

It is not at all an anomaly for fatal pneumonia to follow coronavirus infections.[447] Indeed, historical data support a correlation between pandemic and bacterial pneumonia. It is thought that the majority of deaths in the 1918-1919 pandemic "likely resulted directly from secondary bacterial pneumonia caused by common upper respiratory-tract bacteria." [448] Histopathology of lung tissue sections from that time reveal, "in virtually all cases, compelling histologic evidence of severe acute bacterial pneumonia, either as the predominant pathology or in conjunction [with influenza]." Histological evidence revealed presence of bacterial pneumonia, including bronchopneumonia. Lobar consolidation characteristic of pneumococcal pneumonia, as well as pathognomonic characteristics of streptococcal and staphylococcal pneumoniae were found. In fact, there were no negative lung culture results in any of the specimens. "Bacteria were commonly observed in the sections, often in massive numbers." In fact the bacterial damage was extensive. Vasculitis, capillary thrombosis and necrosis surrounding areas of bronchiolar damage were found. And "without this secondary bacterial pneumonia, experts generally believed that most patients would have recovered."[449]

Interestingly the above-cited paper that found a majority of 1918-1919 pandemic deaths to be from bacterial pneumonia was co-authored by Anthony Fauci, MD who has been tasked with advising the US on proper response to the 2020 COVID-19 pandemic, yet he has not publicly discussed this precedented risk of bacterial pneumonia in 2020, even having performed extensive research himself. It is also known that the 1918-1919 pandemic was the last time that human societies experimented with widespread long-term masking. As now, healthy people were made to wear masks, and it is thought by some that there would have been no pandemic in 1918 without masking. Are we repeating known mistakes from our history and what are the consequences?

The cities of Stockton CA and Boston MA were compared as follows during that pandemic.[450]

"**Masks:** The wearing of proper masks in a proper manner should be made compulsory in hospitals and for all who are directly exposed to infection. It should be made compulsory for barbers, dentists, etc. The evidence before the committee as to beneficial results consequent upon the enforced wearing of masks by the entire population at all times was contradictory, and it has not encouraged the committee to suggest the general adoption of the practice. Persons who desire to wear masks, however, in their own interests, should be instructed as to how to make and wear proper masks, and encouraged to do so.

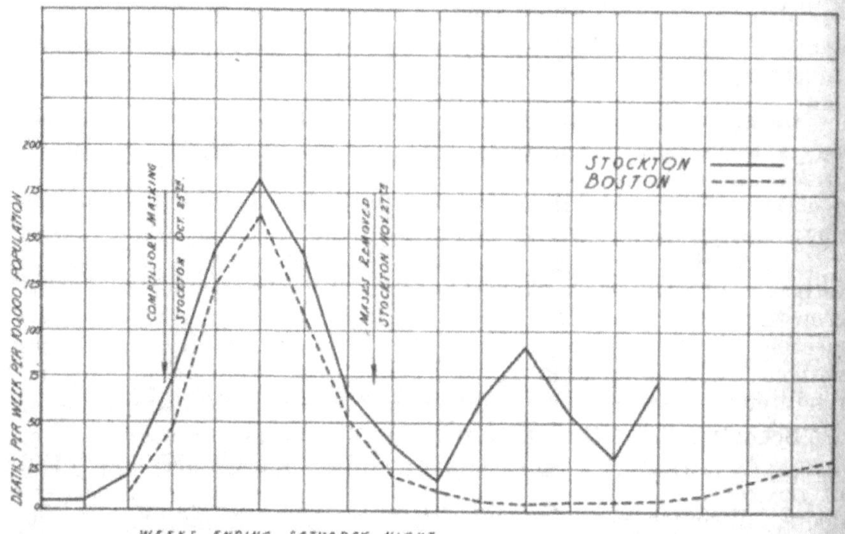

FIG. 17. Stockton, California, and Boston, Massachusetts. Comparative death rates per 100,000 population, by weeks. The use of masks was made compulsory in Stockton, but not in Boston.

One historian writes, "The quarantine, isolation and mask-wearing failed to diminish the spread of the influenza. Instead the practices likely increased fatality and had disastrous economic consequences. The medical policy of 1918 was contrary to the medical science of 1918, and the destructive practices of quarantine, isolation and mask-wearing were largely abandoned."[451]

The harm extended to the next generation. Subsequent health outcomes included increased prevalence of heart disease in infants born in 1919. [452]

Microbial contamination of and from masks

Bacteria are on average ten times the size of viruses, particularly coronaviruses, and have less penetration through masks.[453] Therefore, at least part of the re-circulated flow of bacteria in aerosolized and droplet exhalation does not escape the vicinity of the oral and nasal environment. Bacteria and other microbes are not only retained in this space, but masks themselves are warm, moist repositories of these microbes.

Laboratory testing of used masks from 20 train commuters revealed that 11 of the 20 masks tested contained over 100,000 bacterial colonies. Molds and yeasts were also found. Three of the masks contained more than one million bacterial colonies.[454] Because such particles have been cultured from masks, they are expected to remain fully available to the airways while a mask is worn.

The outside surfaces of surgical masks were found to have high levels of the following microbes, even in hospitals, more concentrated on the outside of masks than in the environment.[455] Staphylococcus species (57%) and Pseudomonas spp (38%) were predominant among bacteria, and Penicillium spp (39%) and Aspergillus spp. (31%) were the predominant fungi. These correlated with the same bacteria and fungi found in samples of the ambient air where the masks were worn.[456]

Evidence is still not abundant of injury from mask-carried microbes due to the experimental and newly adopted practice of widespread masking. Even in Asia, where public use of masks had been more common than in the west, masks were generally only worn by those who had to travel in public while suffering a respiratory illness or those suffering from seasonal pollen allergies. Without regard to the 1918-1919 epidemic, widespread masking is new again in 2020.

We further demonstrate absence of evidence is not evidence of absence. Decades of clinical evidence have attributed a variety of moderate and severe pathologies to microbes that originate in the mouth and nose, as we discuss in this paper.

The mechanism of pathology originating from masks is likely as follows: Microbe-carrying droplets, trapped in masks, stay damp while the mask is worn, whereas without a mask, exhaled droplets and aerosol are known to dry quickly. In the continually damp environment of the mask, bacteria start to proliferate, are re-inhaled and then transferred throughout the body, as discussed below.

Bacteria are exhaled through masks at an increasing rate over the time of use.[457] Outward penetration of masks by bacteria is made worse by the plosive force of coughing, sneezing and talking loudly. Scatter mechanics from the mesh of the mask and resulting chaotic collisions of aerosolized droplets in turn produce a wider contaminated airspace outside the masked mouth than outside the unmasked mouth, in the same way that a screen placed under a faucet disperses the water falling through it.

Cloth mask wearers had significantly higher influenza-like illness when compared to unmasked.[458] This meta-analysis found no benefit of masks against transmission of laboratory-confirmed influenza, in analysis of 14 randomized controlled trials.[459]

James Meehan MD reports seeing patients clinically that have facial rashes, fungal infections, bacterial infections. "Reports coming from my colleagues from all over the world, are suggesting that the bacterial pneumonias are on the rise." Dr. Meehan reports that this is "because untrained members of the public are wearing medical masks repeatedly . . . in a non-sterile fashion."[460]

Recently, a group A strep throat outbreak of unusual size in Michigan public schools where masks are mandatory was reported during the week before this writing.[461] A number of factors may be involved in this outbreak. Not only are students being forced to wear masks, but also schools were closed during lockdown long enough to possibly allow buildup of microbes in their ventilation systems. The problem may be compounded by masks damaging immunity, not being properly washed, poor training of PPE use, or even trapping Streptococcus while forcibly trying to inhale and exhale. After all, deeper inhalation, as we know happens with mask wearing, could have produced a concerning health hazard.

What may be an even more intractable health hazard is the vast range of possibilities where normally colonized strains of oral and nasal bacteria interact with newer virulent strains in the favorable incubating environment of face masks. The possibility of superstrains and their consequences in the population will likely eclipse the effects and the incidence of the relatively mild COVID-19 virus (estimated IFR 0.015[462]), as we have seen from the autopsies discussed above of the 1918-1919 pandemic victims.

Respiratory diseases from oral bacteria

CPAP has been used for decades, but universal masking is very new. We know that wearing the CPAP mask has led to life-threatening Legionella pneumonia as well as Streptococcus infections.[463] This disproves the hypothesis that microbial growth on masks is always benign.

Aspiration pneumonia is a consequence of oral bacteria aspirated into the lungs. The teeth and gums are reservoirs for respiratory pathogens.[464] [465] Oral dysbiosis is a disordered ecosystem of commensal as well as pathogenic bacteria in the mouth. Dental caries and periodontal disease are common results of such dysbiosis. One dental practice estimates that 50% of their patients are suffering from mask-induced dental problems, including decaying teeth, receding gum lines and "seriously sour breath."[466] The dentists theorize that these new oral infections are mostly caused by the tendency for people to mouth-breathe while wearing a mask, which is not consistent with the evolution of the form and functionality of the airways of humans or any other species.

The oral flora is known to comprise over 700 bacterial species, inhabiting the epithelial debris, nutrients and oral secretions in the oral environment. Streptococci, lactobacilli and staphylococci are among the most common of these bacteria. Together, they comprise the biofilm that coats the surfaces of the oral cavity. Clearly, the bacteria benefit from the host, but the host may also benefit from the bacteria and contribute to our immunity by the production of secretory antibodies against new pathogens. The commensal relationship of oral flora with the host is generally benign and stable, unless the same bacteria achieve access to deeper tissues and blood. A number of serious and life-threatening diseases result when this happens.

Bacteria that live in the mouth and upper respiratory tract may be aspirated and cause infection in the lungs. We know that mask-wearers have greater inspiratory flow than non-mask wearers.[467] This is presumably due to the hypoxic condition of mask obstruction to the airways. As a result, microbes may be more likely to be aspirated while wearing a mask than not wearing one.

Damage to the airways results from bacterial colonization. When bacteria localize to the site(s) of infections in the respiratory tract and induce local airway inflammation, epithelial damage results. Such damage only requires bacterial colonization of the airways to begin this process, and to progress to bacterial-induced chronic airway inflammation.[468] This process begins with resident bacteria in oral secretions being aspirated and then adhering to the respiratory epithelium. These stimulate cytokine production and inflammation.[469]

In fact, the very same periodontopathic bacteria are involved in the pathogenesis of respiratory diseases. These may be some of the diseases implicated in COVID-19.[470] Conversely, oral hygiene measures have correlated with improved outcomes in pneumonia patients[471] and those generally with respiratory tract infections, [472] as well as other lung diseases, such as COPD.[473]

Infections don't only take hold from one species of pathogenic microbes. A pathogenic synergy can result in the flourishing of a particular pathogen. This was found to be the case with Aggregatibacter actinomycetemcomitans together with Streptococcus gordonii, both of which are commonly found in the mouth and in its abscesses.[474] With the concentration and culturing of microbes on the surface of a mask, is this pathogenic synergy made more likely while wearing a mask?

Systemic diseases from oral and nasal bacteria

When oral bacteria gain access to blood and deep tissues, they may cause pneumonia, abscesses in lung tissue, subacute bacterial endocarditis, sepsis and meningitis. [475] It is important to consider that endocarditis can be a lifelong infection. Strep pyogenes bacteria has been observed for decades to cause irreversible fibrosis in heart tissue long after the bacteria were no longer found.[476] This bacteria is known by many as "flesh eating strep". Former Streptococcus infections that had seemingly resolved a long time ago may still be positive in an Antistreptolysin O test. For years afterward, flares of toxins can be released in the body at times of stress or secondary infection and cause debilitating symptoms.

Additionally Type 2 diabetes, hypertension, and cardiovascular diseases have been the result of oral bacteria gaining access to deeper tissue.[477] These are among the diseases reported as co-morbidities associated with an increased risk of death attributed to COVID-19. COPD[478] and in this enormous study, cancer can also result simply from the access of oral bacteria to deeper tissue.[479]

Immune-mediated inflammatory disorders, commonly known as auto-immune diseases are correlated with oral dysbiosis. We know that transient bacteria from an oral infection or a dental procedure can gain access to the blood for systemic circulation. Those bacteria can produce toxins that trigger tissue damage or other pathological changes. These molecules may react with antibodies that produce large complexes, which are associated with acute and chronic inflammatory changes.[480] [481] Such auto-immune diseases as rheumatoid arthritis, systemic lupus erythematosus and Sjogren's syndrome all have features of oral dysbiosis.[482]

Autoimmune encephalitis occurs when microbes access brain tissue, triggering neurological or psychiatric symptoms. This complex of diseases include basal ganglia encephalitis, and can be triggered by bacterial, viral and fungal infections. Some of the most pernicious of this group of diseases is pediatric autoimmune neuropsychiatric disorders associated with streptococcal infections (PANDAS). Group A Streptococcus (GAS) is a very common illness, and the most common bacterial infectious agent of sore throat, "strep throat," and is one of the microbial agents involved in PANDAS. GAS causes one million to 2.6 million cases of strep throat each year.[483]

Repeated infections in the nasal cavity can lead to Th1 and Th17 lymphocytes in the surrounding nasal tissue. These are pro-inflammatory and target host cells in a misdirected immune response. The Th17 cells travel into the brain along the olfactory nerves, through the cribriform plate from the nose or throat or palate and into the brain. These in turn stimulate cytokines, which then stimulate microglia. The endothelial cells in the blood brain barrier are broken down by damaging both the tight junctions in the endothelium, and by increasing transcytosis of auto-antibodies that are circulating in the blood to access the brain. This mechanism has been shown to lead to the abrupt onset of neurological and psychiatric symptoms associated with the PANDAS diagnosis.[484]

Our nasal passages are colonized by Staphylococcus bacteria, among other organisms. Under typical circumstances, these pose no threat to the individual; however, Mayo Clinic has warned, (although this statement has now been erased from their site):

> *"A growing number of otherwise healthy people are developing life-threatening staph infections because of mask wearing."*[485]

One of the risks of mask wearing is that masks maintain bacteria in greater numbers and for a longer period of time. This increases the risk of those bacteria entering the respiratory system and/or blood stream through micro wounds.

The following are some of the diseases and conditions that may result. Bacteremia is a condition in which bacteria can travel to internal organs, muscle, bone and prosthetic devices. Toxic shock syndrome is a condition in which some strains of Staphylococcus produce toxins that create high fever, nausea, vomiting and other symptoms. Septic arthritis occurs when staph bacteria infect the joints, which may result in pain, swelling and fever.

The risk of pericarditis caused by staphylococcus has been known since at least 1945.[486] This life-threatening disease has been treated with prolonged antibiotic therapy and aggressive drainage of the pericardium,[487] and, in severe cases, surgical resection of the pericardium.[488] Purulent pericarditis is the most serious consequence of bacterial pericarditis, and is always fatal if untreated. Even in treated patients the mortality rate is 40%.[489]

Streptococcus is a commensal organism of the oral mucosa, and is the most common infective agent causing endocarditis.[490] It is not so unusual for oral Streptococci to gain access to the bloodstream, and oral Streptococci comprise more than half of colonies cultured from blood following dental procedures. "Oral streptococcal bacteremia is frequently associated with the development of septic shock and death."[491]

Cardiovascular and rheumatological outcomes from mask-wearing are unlikely to be realized in the United States for at least several months due to the recentness of mask wearing; although we can learn from the history of prevalence of cardiovascular disease many years after the 1918-1919 forced masking pandemic described previously. These are enormous concerns on the horizon for future public health considerations.

Oral bacteria, with added color, under scanning electron microscope.
https://www.dailymail.co.uk/sciencetech/article-3549713

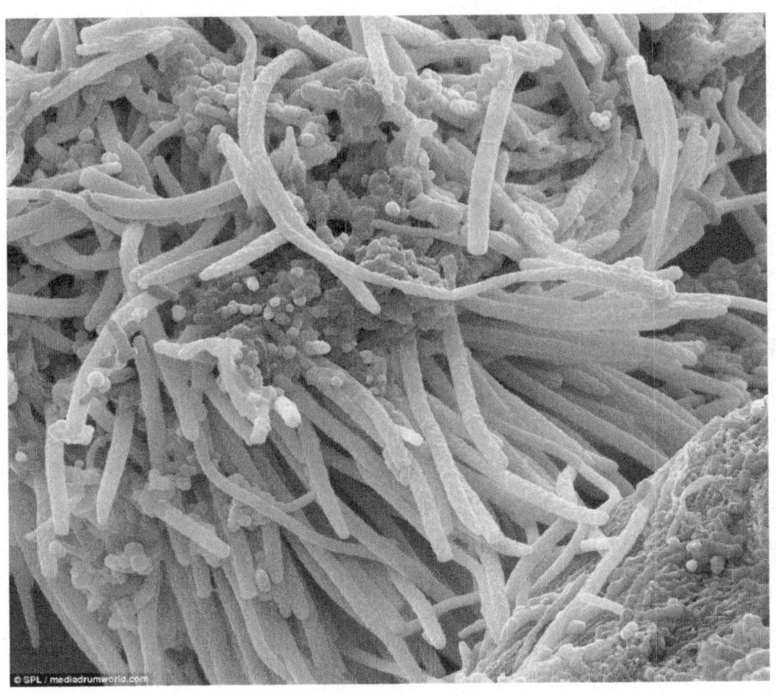

Infections involving fungi, yeast and molds

Aspergillosis is an infection of the lungs by the spores of the Aspergillus fumigatus fungus. These spores are ubiquitous in the environment, indoors and outdoors, and are usually harmless. There are many environmental sources of Aspergillus. Decaying leaves and compost in the outdoors around trees and plants, as well as indoors in bathrooms are common locations of Aspergillus. These spores may be inhaled by those with weakened immune systems and can be a cause or a result of bronchiectasis.[492] This is a chronic airway infection syndrome, and as indicated above, a risk from inhaled fibers. Fungal fibers may be inhaled and accumulate as fungal balls known as aspergillomas. At its worst, Aspergillosis can proceed to systemic infection, with consequences to the brain, heart and kidneys. Invasive aspergillosis spreads rapidly and may be fatal.

Aspergillus as well as candida also produce gliotoxins, which are immunosuppressive toxins that in turn enable proliferation of candida. The mechanism of immunosuppression appears to be by alteration of the structure and function of PMN neutrophils.[493]

It is possible that a warm moist environment, such as a mask worn outdoors or in bathrooms may pick up and harbor fungal spores as well as particulate and/or loose fibers. This is normally not a concern for a healthy person or an unmasked person. When mold spores are inhaled by a healthy person, immune system cells surround and destroy them. Masks provide an alternative environment whereby mold and fungi are held and trapped beyond typical airborne levels. When maintained over the airways, this can create a risk for the mask-wearer. Simply, if the masks retain fungal spores, these may be dislodged with inhalation.

Conclusion

Masks have been shown consistently over time and throughout the world to have no significant preventative impact against any known pathogenic microbes. Specifically, regarding COVID-19, we have shown in this paper that mask use is not correlated with lower death rates nor with lower positive PCR tests.

Masks have also been demonstrated historically to contribute to increased infections within the respiratory tract. We have examined the common occurrence of oral and nasal pathogens accessing deeper tissues and blood, and potential consequences of such events. We have demonstrated from the clinical and historical data cited herein, we conclude the use of face masks will contribute to far more morbidity and mortality than has occurred due to COVID-19.

PDMJ

Masks, false safety and real dangers, Part 3: Hypoxia, hypercapnia and physiological effects

November 2, 2020.
Completed peer-review and revised, November 9, 2020

Boris Borovoy,[x] Colleen Huber,[xi] Maria Crisler[xii]

https://pdmj.org/papers/masks_false_safety_and_real_dangers_part3/

Abstract

Wearing a mask causes physiological changes to multiple organ systems, including the brain, the heart, the lungs, the kidneys and the immune system. We examine changes in oxygen and carbon dioxide concentrations in masked airspace that is available to the airways over the first 45 seconds of wear. Our findings of reduced oxygen and

---

[x] Boris A Borovoy, MPH has a Master in Public Health from Moscow Medical Academy.

[xi] Colleen Huber, NMD is a Naturopathic Medical Doctor and Naturopathic Oncologist (FNORI), writing on topics of masks, COVID-19, cancer and nutrition.

[xii] Maria Crisler is a microbiologist.

increased carbon dioxide in a masked airspace are not inconsistent with previously reported data. We also consider the range of injuries known to occur to the above-named organ systems in a state of hypoxia and hypercapnia. As an excretory pathway, carbon dioxide release by cells throughout the body, and then past the alveoli and then the airways and orifices, has not been previously challenged by deliberate obstruction in the history of the animal kingdom, except for relatively rare human experiments. Self-deprivation of oxygen is also unknown in the animal kingdom, and rarely attempted by humans. We examine the physiological consequences of this experiment.

MASKS and HYPERCAPNIA

Do masks cause systemic hypercapnia?

Airway obstruction is a long recognized cause of retention of carbon dioxide and respiratory acidosis. A sustained level of increased carbon dioxide stays inside of masked air, compared to room air, which in turn sustains a low level of hypercapnia. Rebreathing of exhaled air has been found to quickly elevate [CO_2] in available air above 5000 ppm, and to increase arterial CO_2 concentration and to increase acidosis.[494] The mechanism of mask-induced hypercapnia may also include the moisture on a mask trapping carbon dioxide from exhalation. Some carbon dioxide diffuses in the air, more so if dry, but some portion of it, trapped by water vapor and mask moisture, would form a weak, unstable acid with water, for re-circulation to the airways and lungs. The mechanism is that retention of CO_2 causes an increase in PCO_2. This is the primary disturbance in respiratory acidosis. It results in an increased concentration of both HCO_3^- and H^+, which is measured as a lower pH.

Masks increase respiratory drive and bronchodilation in mild hypercapnia, from sensitive chemoreceptors picking up changes in pH of cerebrospinal fluid. Ultimately in severe hypercapnia, respiratory drive is actually depressed.

Hypercapnia is widely recognized to be an independent risk factor for death. [495] [496] [497] [498] A number of organ systems are negatively impacted, including the brain, heart, lungs, immune system and musculoskeletal system. [499] [500]

How quickly do masks increase carbon dioxide in the masked airspace?

We used a new calibrated carbon dioxide meter to measure ambient carbon dioxide in room air, and then inside the masked airspace of three different masks after donning each in turn. This experiment involved a disposable surgical mask, a N-95 mask and a cloth mask. We recorded carbon dioxide parts per million inside the masked airspace. The meter refreshed its readings at 5-second intervals, and we used those same intervals in recording CO2 parts per million. The maximum CO2 reading on the meter is 10,000 parts per million.

The table of those values are shown in Table 1, with the mean values shown for each 5-second interval in the first 45 seconds. After 45 seconds, the readings passed the maximum meter reading of 10,000 ppm [CO2], and were thereafter indeterminate from the meter.

[For purposes of formatting the book The Defeat of COVID, some intermediate intervals have been deleted.]

Table 1: Measured [CO2] in masked airspace

	Room air	15 sec	30 sec	45 sec	60 sec	75 sec	90 sec
Surgi-cal mask	1072	2256	3306	3074	3378	5483	7472
	1022	1667	3526	6479	7755	9964	>10000
	1074	2400	2948	4794	5994	8095	>10000
	1089	3090	9381	>10000			
	989	3257	6764	9465	>10000		
	1026	3392	6263	>10000			
Mean	1045.3	2677.0	5364.7	7302.0			
N-95	1050	2518	4689	7042	9684	>10000	
	1037	4133	5394	9082	>10000		
	1049	1800	6346	6563	>10000		
	1083	3312	4140	5692	7855	>10000	
	1073	2621	5629	7279	9240	>10000	
	1033	1926	4371	8921	>10000		
Mean	1054.2	2718.3	5094.8	7429.8			
Cloth mask	1084	2218	4914	6494	8410	>10000	
	1066	2467	8480	>10000			
	1050	3573	5768	8966	>10000		
	1062	4129	>10000				
	1051	2301	8555	>10000			
	1044	2772	5149	7385	9260	>10000	
Mean	1059.5	2910.0	7144.3	8807.5			

If we look at the time in which our readings did not yet exceed the maximum of the meter, then we have the following graph, Graph 1, of the average rise in carbon dioxide concentration inside the masked air for each mask, as [CO2] rose over the first 45 seconds of wear.

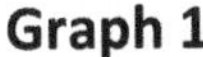

Graph 1

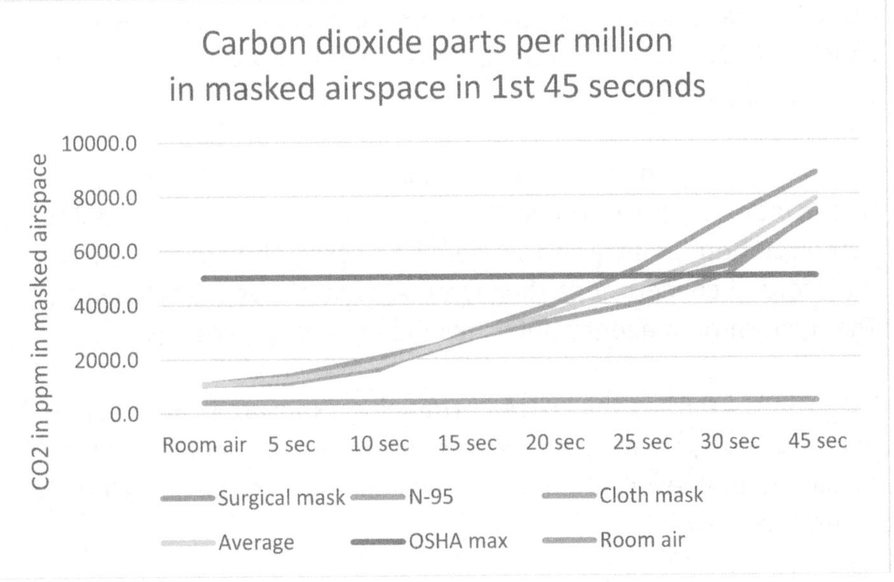

The blue horizontal line in Graph 1 represents the maximum allowable average CO2 concentration in workspace air during an 8-hour work shift, by the Occupational Safety and Health Administration (OSHA) of the US Department of Labor.[501] The green horizontal line represents typical [CO2] in room air, which is 400 parts per million.

After donning each mask, we see that [CO2] in the masked airspace rose above acceptable OSHA limits within the first 30 seconds.

The concentration of carbon dioxide rises similarly during the time of wearing each kind of mask. These findings are consistent with known data on the carbon dioxide concentration of available airspace inside of a mask.[502]

Industrial workspace standards established by OSHA for carbon dioxide concentration in the workspace are for ambient room air, and these have been established since 1979. It is not the case that OSHA has mandated specific CO2 concentrations for masked airspace. However, we examine these standards for available room air, and compare masked airspace to them, because in both cases we may consider [CO2] concentration in the air that is available to the airways and the lungs.

The Food Safety and Inspection Service of the United States Department of Agriculture notes that carbon dioxide gas is used to euthanize both poultry and swine.[503] Concentration of this gas is therefore of concern regarding the use of masks by human beings. That government agency publishes the following warnings:

5,000 ppm = 0.5% is the OSHA Permissible Exposure Limit (PEL) for 8-hour exposure, [504] averaged over the workday. Each of our masks surpassed that level within the masked airspace in the first 25 to 30 seconds of wear.

At 10,000 ppm of short exposure, OSHA says there are typically no effects, possible drowsiness.

At 20,000 ppm, the Food Safety and Inspection Service advises: "Do not enter areas where CO2 levels exceed 20,000 ppm until ventilation has been provided to bring the concentration down to safe levels." We should remember here that each of the masks we studied rose to half of this concentration within the first minute alone.

At 30,000 ppm = 3% [CO2], there is "moderate respiratory stimulation and increased heart rate and blood pressure."

At 40,000 ppm = 4%, OSHA finds [CO2] to be "immediately dangerous to life or health." [505]

Hypercapnia is known to rapidly cause intracellular acidosis in all cells in the body. There is no way to wall off the damage to only affect the lungs, due to constant gas exchange. That is, there is no known way to restrict hypercapnic effects to only the lungs.

The effects of hypercapnia progress in this order: Compensatory attempt at respiratory ventilation, labored breathing, hyperpnea; nervous system changes with changes in motor skills, visual acuity, judgment and cognition, cerebral vasodilation with increasing pressure inside the skull and headache, stimulation of the sympathetic nervous system, resulting in tachycardia, and finally, in case of extreme hypercapnia, central depression.[506 507]

Hypercapnia effects on the lungs and immune system

Exhaled breath contains about 5% = 50,000 ppm carbon dioxide. This is more than 100 times the average of room air which is about 0.04% [CO2]. Exhaled [CO2] is 10 times the upper limit permitted by OSHA in ambient air. Yet each of us exhales this concentration with every breath. Should we re-breathe our own exhaled breath?

A study of healthy healthcare workers found increased [CO2] and decreased [O2] in the respiratory dead space inside a N95 filtering respirator while walking on a treadmill. Within one hour of use, these were "significantly above and below, respectively, the ambient workplace standards."[508] The exhalation valve of the N95 masks did not significantly change its impact on P(CO2).

Hypercapnia has a number of damaging effects on the lungs. Those effects seem to begin with disruption of Na+-K+-ATPase, which leads to impaired alveolar fluid reabsorption. This results in alveolar edema, which in turn obstructs optimal gas exchange.[509] Hypercapnia also inhibits repair of alveoli by impairing proliferation of alveolar epithelial cells via inhibition of the citric acid cycle and resulting mitochondrial dysfunction.[510]

Cilia are made immotile by hypercapnia, along with mask changes in humidity and temperature in the upper airway. This leads to predisposing mask wearers to lower respiratory tract infections by allowing deep seeding of oropharyngeal flora.[511] The lower respiratory system is usually sterile because of the action of the cilia that escalate debris and microorganisms up toward the orifices. Impairment of this process, such as in hypercapnia, may partly explain a correlation of hypercapnia with increased mortality from pulmonary infections.

Hypercapnia correlates with increased mortality in hospitalized patients with community-acquired pneumonia.[512] This seems to be due to a number of factors, including that hypercapnia inhibits IL-6 and TNF as well as inhibiting immune cell function generally,[513] including alveolar macrophages.[514]

Hypercapnia was found to downregulate genes related to immune response. The researchers that had studied this in depth found that "hypercapnia would suppress airway epithelial innate immune response to microbial pathogens and other inflammatory stimuli."[515] They also found suppressive effects of hypercapnia on macrophage, neutrophil and alveolar epithelial cell functions. Hypercapnia was found to decrease bacterial clearance in rats.[516]

In our previous paper in this series, we found a historical correlation with a hypercapnic practice, specifically mask-wearing, and a severe surge of bacterial pneumonia deaths.[517] This time period was mis-named the Spanish Flu, due to a number of reasons, too extensive for this paper. Dr. Anthony Fauci's research team found that every cadaver exhumed from that time in 1918 – 1919 showed the cause of death was bacterial pneumonia, secondary to typical upper respiratory bacteria.[518]

Common and life-threatening diseases of impeded air flow include both obstructive disorders such as asthma, COPD, bronchiectasis and emphysema, as well as restrictive disorders, such as pneumothorax, atelectasis, respiratory distress syndrome and pulmonary fibrosis.

Hypercapnia effects on the blood

Excess carbon dioxide is buffered exclusively in the intracellular fluid, especially in red blood cells. CO2 crosses cell membranes by diffusion, and combines with water to convert to H+ and HCO3-. The hydrogen is then buffered by intracellular proteins such as hemoglobin and organic phosphates. The price paid by the red blood cells for this buffering is seen in the comparison of normal red blood cells on the left versus the damaged and depleted red blood cells on the right.

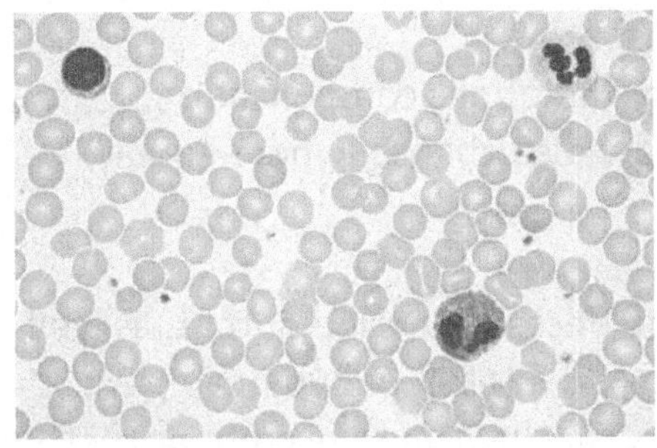

Photo from https://www.flinnsci.com/globalassets/flinn-scientific/all-product-images-rgb-jpegs/ml1297.jpg?v=1bea1f7f72da41ea935dff0a0597f889

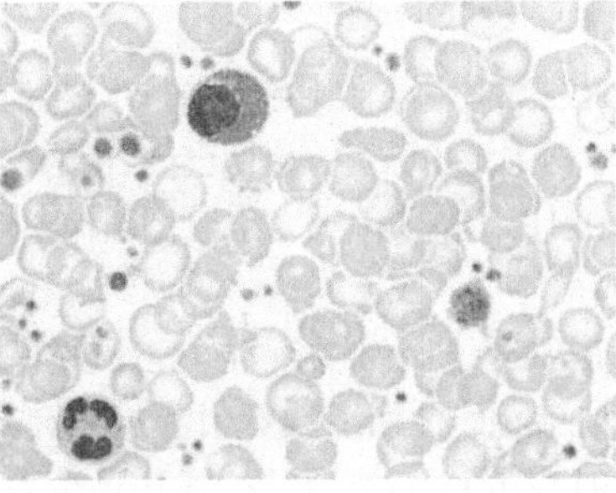

Photo from https://img.medscapestatic.com/pi/meds/ckb/61/36661tn.jpg

The above photo on the right demonstrates secondary polycythemia.. This is a known consequence of hypoxia. This abnormal blood finding may also correlate with dehydration from wearing a mask. The US National Institute of Occupational Safety and Health (NIOSH) says that "particular features of PPE can impose a physiological . . . burden on the healthcare worker." And "dehydration can be a significant problem while wearing PPE."[519] Individuals suffering from dehydration are at risk for relative erythrocytosis, which can manifest as polycythemia vera.[520] Polycythemia vera is an independent risk factor for other cancers, commonly treated with lifelong blood thinning medication. Polycythemia develops slowly over years. Are today's mask wearers at future risk of developing this blood cancer?

Hypercapnia effects on the kidneys

The kidneys are tasked with compensating for the damage inflicted on the blood stream by respiratory acidosis. They must excrete hydrogen ions and reabsorb the newly made HCO_3^-. The Henderson-Hasselbalch equation indicates the extent to which increased HCO_3^- compensates for the acidic condition.

$$pH = pK + \log[HCO_3^-]/(P_{co2})$$

The $[HCO_3^-]$ is a reflection of renal or metabolic compensation, whereas the PCO_2 reflects the primary disturbance, where airway obstruction created an acidemia.[521]

The kidneys show decreased GFR and decreased urine output, as well as increased renal vascular resistance, as a result of hypercapnia.[522] Aciduria increases as a compensatory mechanism to excrete acid. This in turn damages tubules and has been shown to worsen kidney function in those with established chronic diseases.[523]

Hypercapnia effects on the cardiovascular system

A hypercapnic patient may be warm, flushed and tachycardic. A bounding pulse and sweating may also be present. Arrhythmias may be present if there is significant hypoxemia. Arterial pCO_2 above 90 mmHg is not compatible with life, because hypercapnia is necessarily accompanied by hypoxemia, in this case by $pO_2 = 37$.[524] It has been noted that masked patients are often found to be tachycardic, to be discussed more further on in this paper.

Hypercapnia effects on the central nervous system

Central nervous system effects, such as headache, fatigue, dizziness and drowsiness are common effects of chronic obstructive pulmonary disease (COPD),[525] In this patient cohort we also see defects in proprioception, instability of posture and gait, as well as falls, with strong evidence that these result from hypercapnia.[526] There is a progressively increasing sedation from mask use and increased intracranial pressure. Headaches are a common complaint of mask wearers, and are found to be attributable to hypercapnia.[527] Increases in PCO2 lead to increases in cerebral flood flow and cerebral blood volume, as well as a resulting intracranial pressure.[528] These are consistent with findings through the rest of the body.

Slowed performance of reasoning tasks was observed at 20 minutes of inhaling 4.5% to 7.5% [CO2]. [529] When subjects were exposed to 2,500 parts per million carbon dioxide in room air, it was found that their decision-making ability declined by 93%, which was comparable to being drunk or having a head injury.[530] At this same level of [CO2], it was also found that visual performance suffered.[531] We measured this same level of [CO2] inside masked airspace at 15 seconds.

Even smaller CO2 concentrations had deleterious effects. CO2 exposure beginning at 1000 ppm affected cognitive performance, such as problem resolution and decision-making.[532] We measured 1000 ppm [CO2] in masked airspace within the first few seconds of wear.

MASKS and HYPOXIA

Masks create hypoxia in the wearers

A study of 53 surgeons who were non-smokers and without chronic lung disease were shown to have a decrease in saturation of arterial pulsations (SpO2) when performing surgery while masked. Oxygen saturation decreased significantly after the operations in both age groups, with a greater decrease in surgeons over the age of 35.[533]

A study of 39 end-stage renal disease patients wearing N-95 masks for 4 hours during hemodialysis were found to have significantly reduced PaO2 over that time. The average drop in PaO2 was from a baseline PaO2 of 101.7 to 15.8, $p = 0.006$. Respiratory rate increased from 16.8 to 18.8 respirations per minute, $p < 0.001$. Chest discomfort and respiratory distress were also reported by the subjects.[534]

Hypoxia is a health hazard

Hypoxia is deadly. Each year, many workers are injured or die due to oxygen deficiency.[535] "There have been reports of workers who have opened a hatch to an O2-deficient atmosphere and died with only their head inside the hazard. The low level of O2 resulted in a feeling of euphoria and the workers could not comprehend that they only needed to lean back out of the hatch to save their lives."[536]

The issue of mask wearing is especially critical for children. In children, any hypoxic condition is even more of an emergency than it is for an adult. This is partly due to their more horizontal ribs and barrel-shaped chest, resulting in children relying primarily on diaphragm muscles for breathing, not nearly so much intercostal muscles, as in adults. These diaphragm muscles have proportionately fewer type I muscle fibers, resulting in earlier fatigue.[537] Also, a child's tongue is relatively large in proportion to the size of the pharynx, and the epiglottis is floppy.[538] These anatomical differences make a child potentially more vulnerable than an adult to injury from hypoxic assault.

We consider it urgent for children to be released from mask "mandates," based on this information.

Hypoxia in masked airspace

In order to determine the percent of oxygen in masked airspace, we ran 6 trials each for 45 seconds of 3 types of masks: a disposable surgical mask, a N-95 mask and a laundered cloth mask.

We charted the results as follows, showing the average for each type of mask, compared to OSHA workspace requirements for air available to the airways.

Table 2 Measured [O2] in masked airspace

	Room air	5 sec	10 sec	15 sec	30 sec	45 sec	60 sec
Surgical mask	20.9	20.2	19.2	19.1	18.4	18.1	17.7
	20.9	20.1	18.9	18.7	18.1	17.9	17.4
	20.9	20.3	18.7	18.1	17.9	17.6	17.7
	20.9	19.6	19.1	18.7	18.5	17.1	17.5
	20.9	19.8	19.1	18.9	18.7	18.6	16.7
	20.9	20.9	19.0	18.4	18.4	18.2	18.6
Average	20.9	20.2	19.0	18.7	18.3	17.9	17.6
N-95	20.9	20.0	19.1	18.1	18.4	17.2	17.4
	20.9	19.7	19.3	18.5	18.3	18.2	16.7
	20.9	19.6	18.1	18.6	17.8	17.5	17.1
	20.9	20.1	19.4	19.1	18.3	17.2	17.8
	20.9	19.8	19.3	19.0	18.1	18.2	17.4
	20.9	20.9	19.8	18.7	18.1	17.9	17.7
Average	20.9	20.0	19.2	18.7	18.2	17.7	17.4
Cloth mask	20.9	19.6	19.5	17.7	17.5	16.7	17.5
	20.9	20.1	19.2	17.2	17.1	17.0	17.4
	20.9	20.2	19.3	18.4	19.0	17.9	17.1
	20.9	20.0	18.9	18.6	19.3	18.8	18.7
	20.9	20.1	18.4	18.3	17.9	18.1	17.7
	20.9	19.9	18.6	17.8	18.5	19.5	17.1
Average	20.9	20.0	19.0	18.0	18.2	18.0	17.6

Graph 2

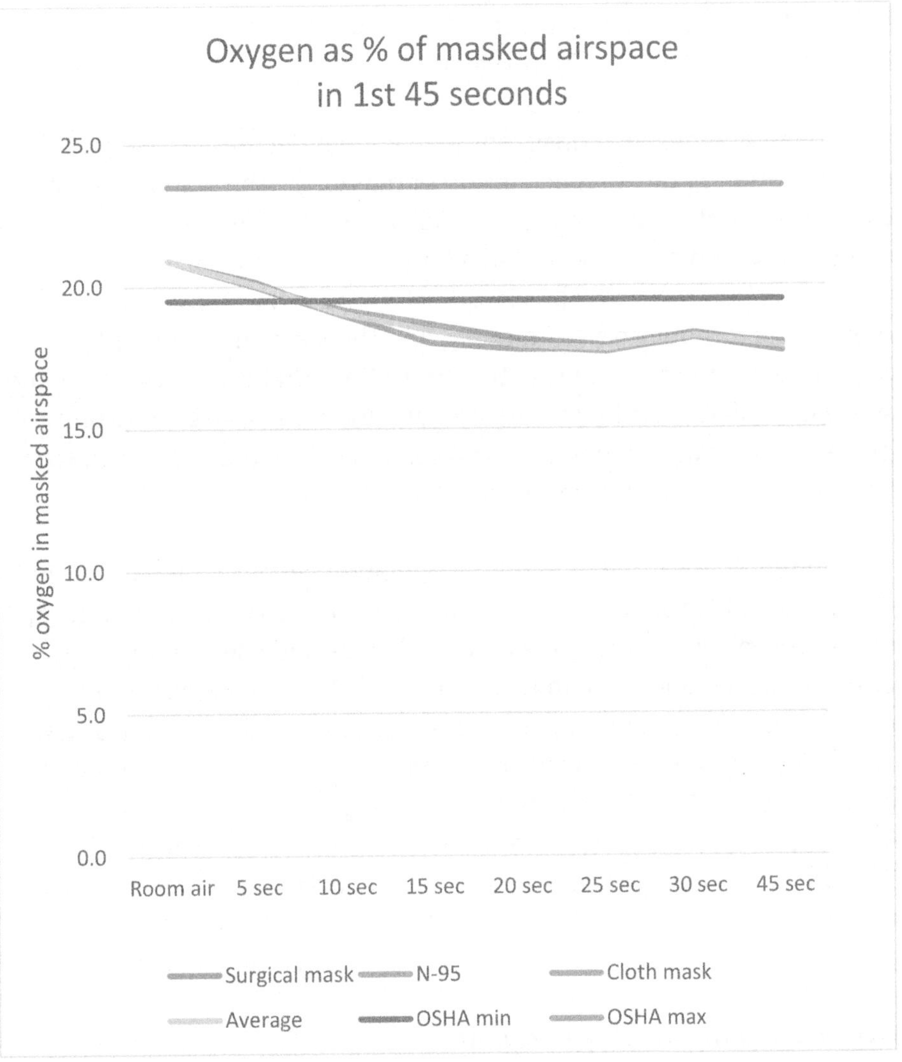

It can be seen from Graph 2 that all of the masks showed similar results, and that in each type of mask, available oxygen as a percentage of available air volume decreased to less than the OSHA required minimum of 19.5%[539] in less than 10 seconds of wear, and stayed below that threshold. Breathing seemed to be shallow until 30 seconds of wear. Then the wearer's responsive drawing of air through pores and side gaps and top gaps around the mask appeared to occur mostly at 30 seconds, but did not compensate adequately to return

[O2] in the masked airspace back above the OSHA minimum requirement of 19.5% [O2] in available air.

The above findings are consistent with known decrease of oxygen concentration in the airspace inside of masks.[540] The standards for oxygen concentration in airspace available to workers has been so strictly enforced by OSHA that in a low-oxygen workspace, employee access must be restricted by using locks or barriers. Oxygen-level monitoring is required before entry, and the space must meet OSHA oxygen-level standards during the entire time that it is in use.[541] Is the space of available airflow to the human airways any less important to protect from low ambient O2, simply because it is the very small space between the mask and the respiratory orifices?

The United States Code of Federal Regulations in paragraph (d) of 29 CFR 1910.134 "requires the employer to evaluate respiratory hazard(s) in the workplace, identify relevant workplace and user factors, and base respirator selection on these factors." This "shall include a reasonable estimate of employee exposures to respiratory hazard(s) . . ." Exceptions are permitted "if the employer can meet the difficult evidentiary burden of showing that the oxygen content can be controlled reliably enough to remain within the ranges specified . . ."[542] Does this leave employers liable for injuries to workers who wear masks?

Hypoxia accompanies hypercapnia

Retention of carbon dioxide reduces oxygen availability, as in COPD. As CO2 builds up in alveoli, the available volume for oxygen in the airspace is reduced. "For each increment in the PaCO2, there will be a more than one-to-one decrease in the PaO2, which will result in severe oxygen deficits, as illustrated in the following graph."[543]

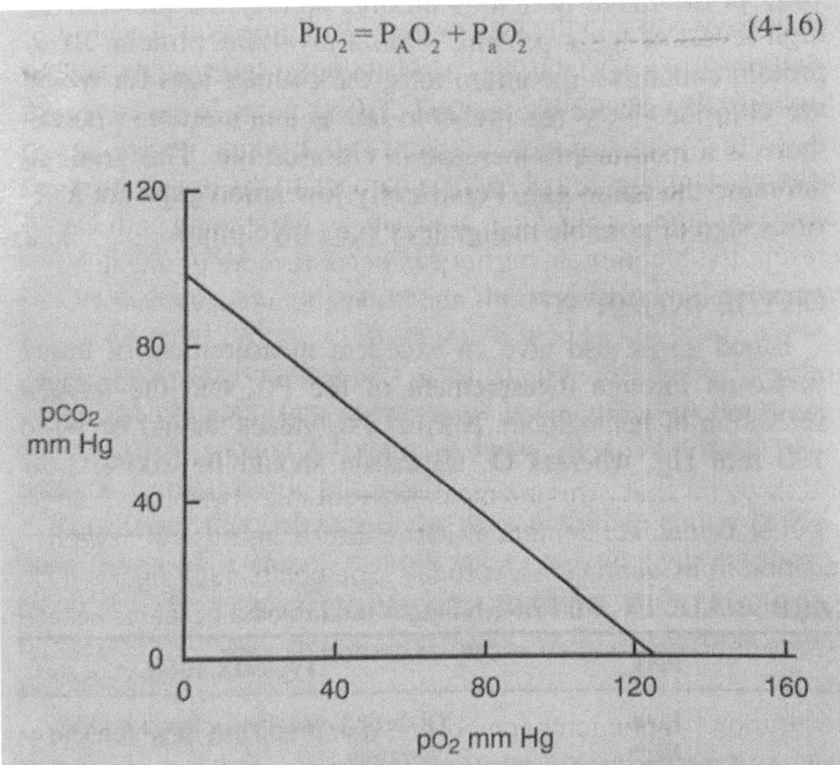

Figure 4–3. The effect of increased Pco_2 on the Po_2 in the alveolus and in arterial blood. This figure demonstrates that as the Pco_2 increases, there is a greater than a one-to-one decrease of Po_2.

From J Henry. Clinical Diagnosis and Management by Laboratory Methods. 19th ed. WB Saunders Co. © 1996.

Hypoxia effects on the brain

Hypoxia, which is the lack of oxygen available to the respiratory system and to the tissues generally, stimulates mitochondria to generate reactive oxygen species (ROS). All body tissues are vulnerable to ROS, but the brain is especially vulnerable. ROS damage lipids, protein and DNA. The brain is 60-70% lipids and low in antioxidants, and is therefore especially vulnerable to ROS damage.[544] For the immature brain, the problem is even worse. Poorly developed scavenging systems and the high availability of free iron leave the child's brain, especially neurons and oligodendrocytes, vulnerable to the oxidative damage of free radicals.[545]

A biochemical mechanism of hypoxia damage to the brain is that hypoxia stimulates a kallikrein – bradykinin – nitric oxide pathway.[546] As a result, the blood-brain barrier can become more permeable. Extravasation of plasma proteins and brain edema may result.[547]

Neurologist and neurophysiologist Dr. Margarite Friesz-Brisson says this about forcing masks on children: "The child needs the brain to learn, and the brain needs oxygen to function. We don't need a clinical study for that. This is simple, indisputable physiology." She warns of a "tsunami of dementia" in the future, because of oxygen deprivation from wearing masks today. She points out long-recognized physiology that re-inhaling our exhaled air creates a state of oxygen deficiency and an excess of carbon dioxide.

Normalization is a phenomenon observed in medicine in which the individual adapts to disadvantageous conditions. Mask wearers may believe that they have become accustomed to wearing a mask. However, the effects of degenerative processes in the brain accumulate during a state of oxygen deprivation. [548]

Cardiovascular effects of hypoxia

It is established that mask wearers work harder at breathing and have greater inspiratory flow than unmasked individuals. This in turn increases sympathetic vasoconstrictor outflow to limb skeletal muscle. After donning a mask, even at rest, mean arterial blood pressure increased by 12 mmHg, and heart rate increased by 27 BPM.[549] Cardiac output is increased and so is prolongation of the QT interval. Vasoactive effects include systemic arterial vasodilation and pulmonary arterial vasoconstriction. It has been found that even at low workloads, in a hypoxic environment, there is not only increased heart rate and blood pressure, but also aortic pressure and left ventricular pressures increase, which in turn promote cardiac overload and coronary demand.[550]

Let us now look at the mechanisms of how this happens. When there is hypoxic assault on the body, hemoglobin is the first sensor. The red blood cells are stimulated to produce nitric oxide, which causes vasodilation and increased blood flow. Hypoxia decreases the threshold needed for this to happen.[551] This vasodilation is a protective effect on the tissues from hypoxic assault, and as a result, the individual becomes tachycardic and agitated.

Hypoxia effects on erythropoiesis

Mask wearing results in loss of available oxygen transport to the tissues. This in turn results in increased erythrocyte production. If hypoxia persists, then free 2,3-DPG is depleted. This leads to increased glycolysis. This leads to production of more 2,3-DPG, which reduces oxygen affinity for hemoglobin. As a result, oxygen is released to the tissues away from vital organs, such as the brain, liver, kidneys and heart. Low oxygenation stimulates production of erythropoietin, which results in more red blood cell production.[552]

Why would we deliberately expose ourselves to persistent hypoxia, which leads to tissue hypoxia in vital organs and increased red blood cell production? Conditions featuring erythroid hyperplasia include but are not limited to: acute myeloid leukemia, congenital dyserythropoietic anemia, microangiopathic hemolytic anemia and sideroblastic anemia.[553] In turn, these can increase risk of polycythemia vera, a disease of thick blood from overproduction of red blood cells. In fact, loss of oxygen is the most common cause of polycythemia vera.[554]

Hypoxia and the gastrointestinal tract

Hypoxia and hypoxia-dependent signaling pathways are becoming better-appreciated in their role in intestinal disease. Tissue hypoxia is recognized as a feature of inflammatory bowel disease.[555] Although intestinal tissue averages 7% [O2], hypoxic stress occurs in infection and inflammation, states which are characterized by oxygen demand being higher than supply. [556] As a result of induced hypoxia, the delicate balance of commensal bacteria on the one hand and limitation of pathogenic bacterial access to tissues on the other is vulnerable to new disruption.

Hypoxia and cancer risk

When there is resistance to inspiratory and expiratory flow, respiratory acidosis and increased lactate levels have been found.[557] At the [O2] levels we measured in the masked airspace, at 17%, higher levels of lactic acid accumulated.[558] This is no surprise given the understanding we have of the metabolic initiation of cancer from Nobel Prize biochemist Otto Warburg. He found that the removal of oxygen initiates the destruction of respiration in cells, and that this process leads to formation of cancer.[559] As tissue oxygenation drops, cells resort to anaerobic glycolysis, which ends the glycolytic pathway with conversion of pyruvate to lactic acid. A marked increase in tissue lactic acidosis results. When oxygen saturation lowers to 30%, blood pH drops to 7.2, which shifts the oxygen-hemoglobin dissociation curve to the right, and sets a vicious cycle in motion, as seen here.

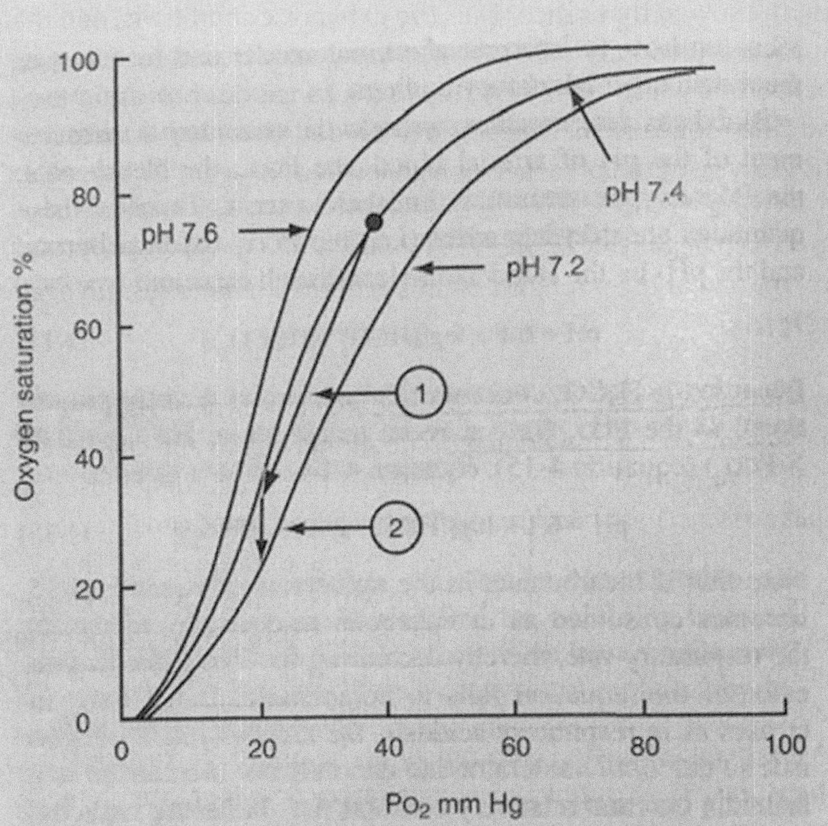

Figure 4–4. The effects of decreasing Po_2 in the allosteric zone of the oxygen-hemoglobin dissociation curve. On the pH 7.4 curve, if the Po_2 drops from 80 to 60, there is little effect on the oxygen saturation. However, a drop from 40 to 20 mm Hg results in a large drop in oxygen saturation from about 80 to 30% (arrow 1 in the figure). With this low oxygen saturation, there is a marked tissue lactic acidosis from anaerobic metabolism. The increased acidosis results in a drop in blood pH to 7.2, shifting the oxygen-hemoglobin dissociation to the right (pH 7.2 curve). Now, for a Po_2 of 30, the oxygen saturation drops even further (arrow 2 in the figure) to about 20%, setting a vicious cycle in motion.

From J Henry. Clinical Diagnosis and Management by Laboratory Methods. 19th ed. WB Saunders Co. © 1996.

Warburg showed that cancer cells live in hypoxic conditions, and that an initial assault on normal cells leads to hypoxia that in turn damages mitochondria, which is the first step in the cancerous process. He found "the root cause of cancer is oxygen deficiency. . . . Cancer cannot survive in the presence of high levels of oxygen."[560]

Hypoxia also negatively impacts the mobility of natural killer cells,[561] which are one of the strongest defenses of the immune system against cancer.

For over a quarter century, Guy Crittenden was editor of HazMat Management, an award-winning occupational health and safety journal. That journal routinely published articles regarding masks and compliance with health and safety laws. He has several major concerns with mask use by the public.[562] One of them is that the disposable surgical masks are sterilized with ethylene oxide, a known carcinogen.[563] Another is that the disposable surgical masks and N-95 respirators are woven with polytetrafluoroethylene (PTFE),[564] [565] PTFE is made using perfluorooctanoic acid (PFOA), a known carcinogen. PFOA has been associated with cancer of the breast,[566] testicles, liver and pancreas.[567] As noted above, inspiratory flow is greater in mask wearers, which brings these compounds deep into the lungs.

Hypoxia and immune function

During a state of hypoxia, the body produces hypoxia-inducible factor-1 (HIF-1). HIF-1 is known to lower T-cell function.[568] CD-4 T-cells have been observed to decline in this process, and they are known to fight viral infections.[569] This raises concerns about whether masks can function as desired during the COVID-19 era. The sudden increase of widespread masking throughout much of the world in 2020 has been motivated by a desire to limit or control the spread of the SARS-CoV-2 virus that is associated with COVID-19. As we have demonstrated, the hypoxia caused by mask-wearing defeats the objective of anti-viral strategy. As we showed in our previous paper in this series, mask use is correlated with higher, not lower, incidence of COVID-19.[570]

Other effects of masks

Masks have been observed to create skin damage in 526 of 542 = 97% of healthcare workers studied. The affected sites were especially the nasal bridge, but also hands, cheeks and forehead. Longer exposure worsened outcome.[571]

US FDA definition of a "medical device"

According to the United States Food and Drug Administration (FDA), a medical device has a specific definition, and it is defined as follows:

> *"An instrument, apparatus, implement, machine, contrivance, implant, in vitro reagent, or other similar or related article, including a component part or accessory which is: recognized in the official National Formulary, or the United States Pharmacopeia, or any supplement to them,*
>
> *-Intended for use in the diagnosis of disease or other conditions, or in the cure, mitigation, treatment, or prevention of disease in man or other animals, or*
>
> *- intended to affect the structure or any function of the body of man or other animals, and which does not achieve its primary intended purposes through chemical action within or on the body of man or other animals and which is not dependent upon being metabolized for the achievement of its primary intended purposes."* [572] [573]

According to the FDA, a prescription for use of a medical device falls to state laws and regulations that determine who can write a prescription for a medical device in each state.[574] The FDA defers to the states regarding who can write a valid prescription. At this time in the United States at least, there are no known prescription rights granted to anyone who does not already hold a license to practice medicine.

However, also in the United States at this time, there are prominent politicians, as well as elected and appointed government leaders, who are "mandating" that citizens in their jurisdictions wear masks when in public.

We submit that a face mask is an apparatus ostensibly intended for prevention of disease, and therefore that it fits within the FDA definition of a medical device, although it is commonly sold over the counter, with no prescription. Therefore, is there now a situation in the United States, and throughout the world, of political leaders prescribing medical devices, including for complete strangers, without so much as a medical consult? Are these same political leaders practicing medicine without a license? If so, are they liable for injuries through these actions, and will they be prosecuted for their actions?

And if these political leaders are prescribing a medical device, without informed consent, then is it also the case that the same politicians and government officials are violating US federal laws regarding informed consent? The US Code of Federal Regulations (CFR) Title 21, Subchapter A, Part 50, Subpart B discusses the requirements of informed consent. Certainly, the same officials are in violation of the Universal Declaration of Human Rights and the Nuremberg Code, which are internationally honored guiding documents on citizens' freedom from medical coercion and medical experimentation.

We therefore urge that people everywhere consider this definition of medical device, and to consider if they want their political leaders and / or their news media to practice medicine on them, without prior medical training, a license to practice medicine, or even so much as an individualized clinical consult.

Conclusion

Our first paper in this series on the false safety and real dangers of masks examined the loose particulate and loose fibers that we found on new masks of various kinds at 40 times and greater magnification, along with the consideration of possible consequences of inhalation of such debris.

Our second paper in this series examined microbial challenges from masks, the dysregulation and imbalance of microbiota in the respiratory tract, and the consequences of such imbalances throughout the body. We showed that face masks are more likely to trap and re-circulate respiratory droplets and microbes, with incubation and proliferation of the same, inside the masked airspace and airways, which increases – not decreases – the risk of infections for major respiratory pathogens, bacterial, fungal and viral.

This paper, the third in our series, focuses on physiological changes induced by hypoxia and hypercapnia. Our findings of reduced oxygen and increased carbon dioxide in a masked airspace are not inconsistent with previously reported data.[575] [576] Evidence of damage to multiple organ systems from the documented levels of [O2] and [CO2] in available airspace between a facemask and the airways are cited above and are abundant in the medical literature.

The pathological triad of micro-particles as long-term hazards, and bacterial and fungal infections as mid-term hazards, as well as injury from hypoxia and hypercapnia in the short-term, are expected to have synergistic results in endangering the health of masked people. Because of the extensive risk to mask wearers documented in these three papers, we urgently recommend that no adult or child be coerced to wear a mask under any circumstances. We further recommend that facemask hazards be published prominently and that masks only be worn by adults who choose to do so, and only with freely given informed consent, with full knowledge of their hazards, and that their use be prohibited for children, adult students and workers.

If on the other hand, widespread use of masks and mandating the same continue, then the question arises, from the data shown herein, whether morbidity and mortality from mask-wearing will exceed those of COVID-19 or other known infectious diseases. What will be the long-term effects of mask wearing if it continues? And will we be able to distinguish mask injury from COVID-19 or other pathologies? The evidence presented here, in summary of clinical data from around the world, show that masks can accelerate morbidity and mortality in those who are already ill, and that masks can sicken healthy people. Before masks are forced onto school children and workers, why are animal studies not being done with all-day masking, to investigate safety issues? How much of an increase in mask-related illnesses will we have to observe before mask "mandates" end?

PDMJ

Masks, false safety and real dangers, Part 4:

Proposed mechanisms by which masks increase risk of COVID-19

December 7, 2020.
Completed peer-review and revised, January 8, 2021

Colleen Huber, NMD [xiii]

https://pdmj.org/papers/masks_false_safety_and_real_dangers_part4/

Abstract

Mask "mandates" in 2020 have resulted in no reductions in incidence of COVID-19, as detected by positive polymerase chain reaction (PCR) tests among nations or US states. Increased rates or insignificant change in incidence of SARS-CoV-2 infections, as detected by PCR tests, have followed mask mandates throughout the world and in US states. Masks are therefore a possible risk factor for infection with SARS-CoV-2 and higher incidence of COVID-19 disease. This paper

[xiii] Colleen Huber, NMD is a Naturopathic Medical Doctor and Naturopathic Oncologist (FNORI), writing on topics of masks, COVID-19, cancer and nutrition.

examines the known physical and chemical attributes of respiration through and involving the periphery of and inside of masks that may lead to a better understanding of the reasons for this phenomenon of increased COVID-19 incidence following mask use.

COVID-19 incidence in masked and unmasked populations

The Council of Foreign Relations surveyed the citizens of 25 countries in mid-July, 2020. Their question was: "Have you always worn a face mask outside the home in the last seven days?" [577] Yes responses ranged from the highest of 93% in Singapore to the lowest of 1% in Finland and Denmark. In our team's research, we examined those same countries 3 months later, in early October 2020, regarding COVID-19 deaths and COVID-19 cases. There seemed to be no clear, identifiable pattern with regard to deaths. However, there was a trend of the countries with the least mask use in July 2020 showing generally fewer COVID-19 cases three months later.[578]

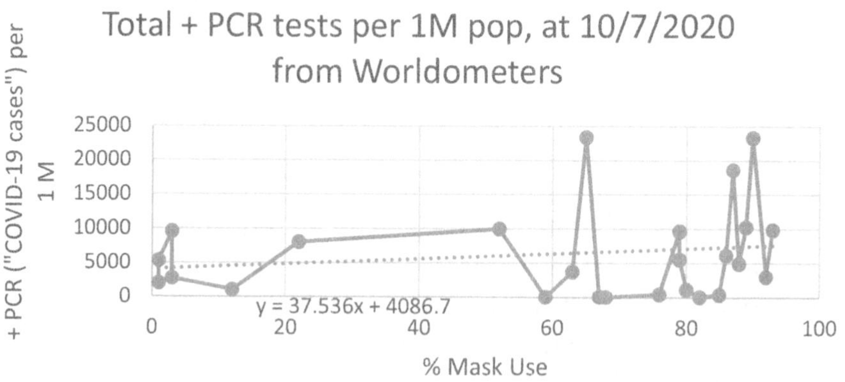

Population data for countries and US states have shown that declared numbers of COVID-19 cases have more often increased than decreased after government "mandates" to their citizens to wear masks in those jurisdictions. Timelines of seven countries, Israel,

Peru, Philippines, Spain, France, Hungary and Argentina, all showed no prompt impact of mask mandates on change in number of cases or hospitalizations from COVID-19.[579] [580] But all seven of those countries showed increases in SARS-CoV-2 cases within 12 weeks following mask mandates. Five US metropolitan areas and six US states were also examined and showed similar patterns of increased reported SARS-CoV-2 cases. The Czech Republic showed sharply increased COVID-19 incidence immediately following that country's second mask mandate. The graphs discussed were prepared using data from the COVID Tracking Project Data Download [581] and from Our World In Data.[582] None except the Czech Republic showed a distinct inflection point from decrease to increase or vice versa of positive PCR tests at the time of, or shortly after, a mask mandate. The trend line of cases and hospitalizations in each jurisdiction generally increased after some weeks following the mandate. All areas showed increases in COVID-19 cases following mask mandates, except for New York City and Mississippi, both of which had already begun a sharp descent in COVID-19 cases for at least two weeks prior to mask mandates and then continued without appreciable change.

The foregoing data from The Covid Tracking Project Data Download, Our World in Data, The Council of Foreign Relations and our research team show higher rates of positive COVID-19 PCR tests in regions that had previous higher mask use.

The largest population-based study of facemasks and COVID-19 outcomes to date, known as the DANMASK-19 or Danish Mask Study, was conducted in April and May, 2020, and was released in mid-November 2020.[583] It enrolled 3030 participants to wear masks, and 2994 to remain unmasked, and for one month followed 4,862 of them who were able to complete the study. For that month, approximately one half of the participants wore masks, and the other half did not, while they went about their daily activities, in a non-lockdown environment. The average amount of time spent outside the home was 4.5 hours per day.

At the end of that month, data was collected on PCR values, IgM and IgG antibodies and / or hospital admission. Missing data and inconclusive results, patient-reported findings on home tests and other variables limited accurate assessment of results. It was found that approximately 2% of each group, 1.8% masked and 2.1% unmasked, were determined to have become infected with SARS-CoV-2. The DANMASK-19 study authors confessed a prior bias in favor of mask use, despite lack of any medical research prior to March 2020 confirming a preventive effect of masks against any viral illnesses. According to the existing research and meta-analyses prior to March 2020, facemasks have never been shown to be effective against transmission of viral infections.[584] [585] [586] Nor have masks been shown to be effective specifically against SARS-CoV-2.[587] The conclusion of the DANMASK-19 study was that masks did not significantly reduce COVID-19 infection rates, and about 0.5% of each group tested positive for other viruses. The DANMASK-19 study found, "A recommendation to wear a surgical mask when outside the home among others did not reduce, at conventional levels of statistical significance, incident SARS-CoV-2 infection compared with no mask recommendation."

The data above show that regions with higher mask use either had higher rates or insignificant change in positive COVID-19 PCR tests. It is the goal of this paper to examine the mechanisms of mask use that may be most likely to give rise to these findings.

Proposed physical mechanisms for increased COVID-19 transmission due to mask use

A 2020 Duke University study included an examination of a cloth masks containment failure. The mesh of certain masks served as a dispersing tool for expired respiratory droplets.[588] Larger exhaled droplets from an unmasked person are known to fall to the ground quickly and at a short distance forward from the mouth.[589] The Duke University study found, however, that the mesh of the mask dispersed larger exhaled respiratory droplets "into a multitude of smaller droplets, . . . which explains the apparent increase in droplet count relative to no mask in that case." Smaller particles were also found to be more likely to stay airborne longer than larger droplets. As a result those particular cloth masks examined in the Duke University study were considered to be "counterproductive."

Aerosolized breath contain particles that can remain airborne for hours. "These time scales vary from many seconds to a few hours in typical indoor settings." [590]

A seldom considered aspect of masking is the nozzle effect. Gaps are present around the edges of all masks except for the most tightly fitted, and therefore possibly most suffocating, respirators. Side gaps and brow gaps around the periphery of a mask are openings by which exhaled and unfiltered aerosol is released into the air. As a stream of fluid (liquid or gas) is forced by exhalation against a constricted opening, both its speed and kinetic energy increase. Bernoulli's equation explains the conservation of energy as a fluid is forced through a narrowed opening:

$$\frac{1}{2}\rho v^2 = \frac{\frac{1}{2}\mathrm{mv2}}{V} = \frac{KE}{V}$$

Where ρ is the fluid density, and the kinetic energy per unit volume KE/V is ½ of mass times the square of velocity per total Volume (V). Compression of exhaled gas inside a mask raises fluid density compared to unmasked airspace. According to Bernoulli's equation above, velocity and kinetic energy as air is expelled would therefore be higher from masked than from unmasked airspace.

Pressure inside masked airspace is also higher, because there is obstruction to release of exhaled air by the mask mesh. Pressure and volume remain inversely proportional in a closed system with no other variables. This is explained by Boyle's Law, which is as follows: P = k/V, where P = pressure, k is a constant and V = volume.

The formula for gas pressure, PV = nRT, where n = the number of moles of gas, R is the universal gas constant and T is Kelvin temperature, also shows why pressure increases inside masked airspace on exhalation. R and T and V all stay fairly constant, but the number of moles of gas increase as the exhaled air, and its principal components (79% nitrogen, 16% oxygen and 4% carbon dioxide) emerge from the lungs. With all other variables held constant in PV = nRT, pressure can be expected to increase inside masked airspace on exhalation as n increases.

These mechanical considerations are applicable to masks in that a mask wraps around the sides of the face, back toward the ears, where only small gaps remain for the unimpeded release of exhaled breath. Similarly, gaps at the contours of the sides of the nose and under the chin leave only narrowed gaps for unfiltered, unobstructed exhalation above and below the mask respectively.

As a result, there are side jets, back jets, a crown jet, brow jets and a downward jet that emerge from the mask in each of those directions. Farther transmission of virus-laden fluid particles have been found from masked individuals than from unmasked individuals, by means of "several leakage jets, including intense backward and downwards jets that may present major hazards," and a "potentially dangerous leakage jet of up to several meters." These masks "have the potential to disperse virus-laden fluid particles by several meters." [591] Backward airflow was found to be strong with all masks and faceshields studied, compared to not masking. Schlieren imaging revealed farther brow jets (upward flow) in surgical masks and cloth masks, 182 mm and 203 mm respectively versus none discernible at all with no mask. With regard to side jets and back jets, the authors found:

> "It is important to be aware of this jet, to avoid a false sense of security that may arise when

standing to the side of, or behind, a person wearing a surgical, or handmade mask or shield."

These jets were shown to contain viral particles measuring from 0.03 to 1 microns when expelled through the side gaps of both N-95 and surgical masks.[592]

Unmasked individuals on the other hand are unlikely to transmit viral particles anywhere near the distance that a masked individual can unwittingly contaminate. Oral microbial flora dispersed by unmasked healthcare workers standing one meter from the workspace failed to contaminate exposed plates on that surface.[593]

A concern arises then regarding the exposure of people who are positioned next to or behind or standing over a masked individual. Whereas unmasked individuals have been shown to have no or short-distance viral transmission, a leakage jet of up to several meters is a condition that makes a masked person a considerably greater risk for aerosol dispersion toward those in the vicinity who may be concerned about their own exposure to SARS-CoV-2 or other respiratory pathogens.

Proposed chemical mechanisms for increased COVID-19 susceptibility due to mask use

Low oxygen has been measured in the airspace inside a variety of masks. Available oxygen as a percentage of available air volume decreased to less than the US Occupational Safety and Health Administration (OSHA) required minimum of 19.5% [594] in less than 10 seconds of wear, and stayed below that threshold.[595] A study of 53 surgeons found a decrease in saturation of arterial pulsations (SpO2) when performing surgery while masked. Oxygen saturation decreased significantly after the operations.[596]

During a state of hypoxia, the body produces hypoxia-inducible factor-1 (HIF-1). HIF-1 is known to lower T-cell function.[597] CD-4 T-cells have been observed to decline in this process. However, it is essential to understand that CD-4 T-cells are known to fight viral infections.[598] This raises concerns that masked persons might more easily acquire, incubate and subsequently transmit a virus that has been the focus of intense attention, fear and concern throughout the world in 2020.

Another effect of HIF-1 is that it reduces angiotensin converting enzyme 2 (ACE2).[599] This enzyme plays key roles in maintaining blood pressure and electrolytes and controlling inflammation. Cells throughout the body carry receptors for ACE2, and they are especially concentrated in lung and bronchial epithelial cells, and also present in oral and nasal mucosa. ACE2 receptors are also the initial portal by which SARS-CoV-2 enter cells of the upper respiratory tract. An effect of SARS-CoV-2 is that it down-regulates ACE2 receptors.[600] A masked person with a new SARS-CoV-2 infection then would lose both ACE2 and ACE2 receptors. ACE2 is helpful to counteract damaging effects of Angiotensin II, such as inflammation and vasoconstriction. But as ACE2 effects on the body plummet from both loss of ACE2 and loss of receptors, the masked person with a new SARS-CoV-2 infection is especially at risk of marked inflammation and accompanying disease severity. So pathogenic effects of SARS-CoV-2 would be augmented by a hypoxic influence, such as masking, and therefore, would be contraindicated in one who could become infected with this coronavirus. Therefore, mask-induced hypoxia may make the difference between an asymptomatic or lightly symptomatic interaction with SARS-CoV-2 in a normoxic individual, compared with a severe case of COVID-19 in a hypoxic individual.

Carbon dioxide has also been found to rise within 30 seconds of donning a mask and remains at high levels in masked airspace, above OSHA requirements.[601] Masked individuals have been found to manifest evidence of hypercapnia,[602] which affects multiple body systems.[603] [604]

Hypercapnia immobilizes cilia, the hair-like structures we rely on to clear pathogens from the upper airways. This leads to predisposing mask wearers to respiratory tract infections and vulnerability to deep entry of pathogens.[605] The lower respiratory system is usually sterile because of the action of the cilia that escalate debris and microorganisms up toward the mouth and nose. Impairment of this process, such as in hypercapnia, is a risk factor for pathogenesis and severity of respiratory infections.

Hypercapnia was found to downregulate genes related to immune response. It was found that "hypercapnia would suppress airway epithelial innate immune response to microbial pathogens and other inflammatory stimuli."[606] Suppressive effects of hypercapnia were found on macrophage, neutrophil and alveolar epithelial cell functions.

Another effect of masks that may have direct impact on vulnerability to COVID-19 infection is that a mask covers some of the small portion of body surface area that would otherwise be exposed to sunlight in winter, when seasonal coronaviruses are most prevalent. Skin exposure to the sun is the initial mechanism for bodily production of vitamin D. Vitamin D is known to interfere with viral replication,[607] [608] and has been particularly essential as prophylaxis against COVID-19 severity.[609]

Conclusion

Population studies show that the use of masks either resulted in an increased incidence of COVID-19 or had no impact. None of the examined jurisdictions experienced decreased incidence of COVID-19 after the introduction of mask mandates, except two that had already begun a sharp descent in COVID-19 cases weeks earlier. Two physical mechanisms are proposed to directly contribute to this finding, based on current available research. The first is scatter mechanics of dispersed respiratory droplets becoming aerosolized on collision with the mesh of a mask on outward exhalation and then lingering in air. The second is the pressurized and distant peripheral jets of unfiltered exhaled aerosol from the nozzled edges of a mask. These phenomena result in viral particles lingering longer and traveling farther in airspace from a masked person than exhaled respiratory droplets falling close to the body from the orifices of an unmasked person. There are also chemical mechanisms for increased COVID-19 cases in masked populations. This is likely due to immune suppression caused by hypoxic and hypercapnic conditions, as well as acidotic, immobilized cilia in the lungs, and reduced skin surface available to sunlight for Vitamin D production. Caution is therefore urged against use of masks among those who wish to reduce the risk, either for themselves or others, of infection with SARS-CoV-2 or COVID-19 disease.

Where my rights end

I don't have unlimited rights with respect to you. How do I know this? Since the signing of the US Constitution and its Amendments, and the Enlightenment generally, but more so since Emancipation, the 19th Amendment, the Voting Rights Act, and the US Civil Rights Movement, the most widely accepted understanding of human rights is that they pertain to the equality, autonomy, dignity, freedom from bondage or oppression and the equal and full exercise of self-determination that contemporary people generally acknowledge as self-evident, and inherent to, and cherished equally in each human being. The above landmark events establish, among other rights, for you to be free from oppression or harm done to you by me or anyone else. Internationally, the Universal Declaration of Human Rights, the Nuremberg Code, the Helsinki Declaration are all guiding documents to governments around the world on the treatment of human beings, and our right as humans to be free from abuse.

This right of the individual to be free from inflicted harm has been widely appreciated, if not so widely upheld, since much earlier in human history. Our human right to be free from injury caused by others is not to be violated by any entity, within the guidelines of The Golden Rule: Do unto others as you would have them do unto you. Rabbi Hillel said the essential and inextricable corollary: "That which is hateful to you, do not do to another. That is the whole of the Torah. All the rest is commentary. Go and study." The Buddha is quoted: "You shouldn't harm others if you love yourself." The Golden Rule is attributed to Jesus in each of the Gospels. The instruction not to inflict harm is so essential that it is basic to major religions. It is the central operating principle of civil societies, and harmonious institutions, alliances, friendships and households. The Golden Rule is the *only* common precept among all the world's religions.

So it is well-established that I am not allowed to cause harm to you. It is worth repeating: I may not hurt you. As a physician, I work under, as the central principle of my philosophy and my practice, the Golden Rule as Hillel's corollary, otherwise known as the Hippocratic Oath: First Do No Harm.

But aren't we all under the same oath? Aren't we all obligated to not cause harm?

I do not ask others to wear a mask. Why? I have no right to obstruct anyone's breathing. I have no right to cause widely demonstrated and clinically confirmed hypoxic injuries to the lungs, brain, heart and musculoskeletal system known in the peer-reviewed research to be caused by masking. Yes, I am sorry that you have been told over the last year that masks don't reduce oxygen, by emphatic and dogmatic people, but the fact remains that oxygen deficit during mask-wearing is very thoroughly established in peer-reviewed clinical data. Here[610], here[611] and here[612], for example. And yes, surgeons also suffer from deoxygenation.[613] Excess of carbon dioxide, as it accumulates inside a mask, also is a mild poisoning of the entire body, and this is also established in clinical data. [614] [615] So if you demand that a child, a worker, a traveler, a consumer or anyone else wear a mask, you have been demanding that they mildly poison themselves. I know this is vexing for some to read, but you cannot inflict harm with any moral authority, and you need to stop that, now that you know it's an assault, if you want to be able to live with yourself, or to exist peacefully with a good conscience.

But what about viruses?

What about them? There are trillions of viruses on our skin.[616] Must all skin be covered? With regard to respiratory viruses, light, airborne, breeze-carried, aerosolized viruses have wafted through the mesh of masks, and shot out the side jets under people's ears so consistently for the last year, that masked populations have had higher rates of COVID-19 than unmasked populations.[617] The 'mask and distance' strategy used over most of the past year has had no positive impact on the epidemic process, either globally or in the US population. Covid has a 99.74% survival rate among even those who take *none* of the best-known measures against it.[618] [619] Well-informed doctors keep our patients stocked with adequate preventive strategies against covid, which have an excellent track record in combination therapy of prevention and recovery,[620] none of which involves the health-destroying practice of mask-wearing. As a physician who has studied covid for about a year, my opinion is that covid is no threat whatsoever to well-informed people in any age group who have access to one or more inexpensive remedies, especially now that it, like all previous coronaviruses, has passed peak virulence and pathogenicity, and has mutated into more benign variants, with rapidly declining hospitalizations.[621]

Why do I have no right to demand that another person wear a mask? Even inside my home? Even when people are only a few feet away from me? Even when we hug or shake hands?

Because I have no right to raise their blood pressure by an average of 12 points systolic.[622] I have no right to force anyone to incubate an average of 100,000 bacterial colonies in their airways or on their skin, which were cultured from the used masks of European train commuters.[623] I have no right to immobilize the cilia of people's airways, which they need to help escalate inhaled viruses, bacteria and fungi up the trachea, away from the lungs.[624] I have no right to put asbestos fiber size particles deep into their lungs, where those are unlikely to be exhaled, and where those particles can begin the process of pulmonary fibrosis (the most frightening and hopeless disease I have seen as a physician).[625] I have no right to interfere with the function of a person's immune system to perform its usual functions.[626] [627] [628]

My research team has compiled the most comprehensive research in the English language on the hazards of masks, through several peer-reviewed articles here,[629] in which we cited and linked to over 200 studies, mostly from the peer-reviewed published medical literature.

I do not have the right to impose a face covering on anyone, to put an obstacle in the path of anyone's breath, and neither does anybody else, ever. If you think that you have that right, to make that demand of others, are you willing to pay the reparations, for both suffering and medical expenses, and higher insurance premiums for all, for the pneumonia, pulmonary fibrosis, cancer, and other diseases and injuries that may result over the coming years from mask-wearing?

Do others have the right to make you wear a mask? Does their fear of a virus take precedence over your right to remain free from mask-induced injuries?

Conclusion

To repeat Dr. Thomas Levy's memorable quote, "There already exist numerous ways to reliably prevent, mitigate, and even cure COVID-19, including in late-stage patients who are already ventilator-dependent." Dr. Levy documents many of them in this paper.[630]

Those who were diagnosed and sickened from the most feared viral pathogen of our time fell into several categories. Either they died from the disease, or they healed from one of the interventions discussed in this book, or fortunately, healed with none of those interventions. The 500+ studies cited in this book amply demonstrate that it was enough that one or the other of the nutrients discussed herein was adequate to prevent or to vanquish COVID-19, without the need to use all of them. Therefore, because any one of these nutrients proved adequate to heal patients to complete recovery, then the patients who succumbed to COVID-19 disease had likely been deficient in all of these nutrients, and a lack of all of these nutrients was likely a necessary condition for pathogenesis of COVID-19.

Because of the therapeutic impact and success that each of the above nutrients have had in reversing the devastation of COVID-19, the case has been amply demonstrated that each of these nutrients must be made available immediately and widely throughout the world, for both preventative and prompt therapeutic uses. Safe and useful pharmaceuticals such as hydroxychloroquine and ivermectin must be available and unrestricted for prescribers and their patients.

There is therefore no need or justification for pandemic status of COVID-19. Furthermore, nutritional interventions, not masks and not lockdowns, should be used without hesitation as first-line treatment, as well as prevention, of COVID-19. In future outbreaks and surges of infectious pathogens, the information presented in this book should be considered first in the decision-making process, from the level of the individual and the household to the medical community and governments.

About the Author

Colleen Huber NMD is a Naturopathic Medical Doctor in Tempe, Arizona. She was the Keynote Speaker at the 2015 Euro Cancer Summit. Dr. Huber is President of the Naturopathic Cancer Society. She is a Naturopathic Oncologist and Fellow of the Naturopathic Oncology Research Institute. She authored the largest and longest study in medical history on sugar intake in cancer patients in 2014. Her other writing includes her books Manifesto for a Cancer Patient and Choose Your Foods Like Your Life Depends On Them, and she has been featured in the books America's Best Cancer Doctors and Defeat Cancer. Her academic writing has appeared in The Lancet and Cancer Strategies Journal, and other medical journals. Her research interests have been in nutrition and the use of therapeutic approaches targeting metabolic aspects of cancer. Since the spring of 2020, Dr. Huber's research interests have focused on the health hazards of masks and lockdowns. Most of these peer-reviewed articles are in Primary Doctor Medical Journal, https://PDMJ.org.

Glossary

The human immune system is vastly more complex than this brief glossary explains, but it should help orient the reader who is unfamiliar with immunology to some of the basic players in the innate and adaptive immune systems. The cells described below may be seen as specialized soldiers in the body's war against invading microbes. They are coordinated and synergistic in their activities. Other analogous imagery may involve the specialized players in team sports such as baseball.

However, it may be most appropriate to view the following components of the immune system as tools in a workshop. Your immune system uses these tools carefully, devastatingly and synergistically against arriving pathogens. The treatments discussed in this book are indisputably lifesaving, and when taken by a person with symptoms, they leave SARS-CoV-2 in its true role as merely the nuisance of the common cold. The immune system is even more essential. We would be in mortal peril without our immune systems, unable to survive any infection, and would certainly die within days.

The players (or tools) of the human immune system are as follows, in these two broad interacting divisions:

The innate immune system consists of the first responders. These are:

1) Epithelial barrier: The skin is our first defense against invading pathogens. We are vulnerable when it is lacerated, punctured or abraded. Mucous membranes lining the respiratory and gastrointestinal tracts encounter invading pathogens with a variety of defenses, such as cilia in the upper airways.
2) Mast cells
3) Phagocytes, such as macrophages and neutrophils
4) Monocytes, which are immature macrophages
5) Dendritic cells and other antigen-presenting cells
6) Cytokines, such as interferons and interleukins
7) Natural killer cells
8) Complement

The adaptive immune system consists of cells that have been trained by the innate immune system in more specialized tactics against specific pathogens. They are slower to respond because of this training, but more specifically targeted to the invading pathogens. The adaptive immune system consists of:

1) B-cells, or B-lymphocytes
2) T-cells, or T-lymphocytes

Adaptive immune system: This is the supple, responsive part of our immune system that makes and includes B cells and T cells. It adapts to a new pathogen, and makes antibodies and T-cells, in order to fight this new pathogen more effectively in the future than on first encounter. This branch of the immune system specializes in specificity for known pathogens and the memory needed to recognize them in case of future return.

Antibody (Ab): A protein, also called Immunoglobulin, on the surface of B-cells that was made in response to the presence of a specific non-self-material in the body, an antigen, such as a bacterium or virus. The antibody neutralizes the antigen by binding to it, not letting it reproduce or to infect new cells. Each activated B-cell becomes a plasma cell that makes one unique antibody against one unique antigen.

Antigen: A new protein that arrives to the body. First the innate immune system reacts within the first 12 hours of contact. Then the adaptive immune system within the first 5 days.

Antigen-presenting cells: Cells in our innate immune system that display a foreign protein on their surface. These are specifically and efficiently displayed, via MHC molecules, to T-cells, and often also activate those T-cells.

Autoimmunity, autoimmune disease: An intolerance in the adaptive immune system for one or more of the body's own proteins (self-antigens), which lead to damage to tissues committed by the adaptive immune system. Rheumatoid arthritis, Type I diabetes, multiple sclerosis and lupus are examples.

B-cells: B-cells are activated by the presence of antigens (foreign proteins). They then become plasma cells and produce a high quantity of specific antibodies to a specific antigen, and then they die.

Bone marrow: All blood cells, white and red, in adults originate in the deep interior of bone, the marrow.

Cathelicidins: Proteins made by neutrophils. They are directly toxic to microbes and activate more leukocytes.

CD4+ T-cells: These are helper T-cells that have CD4 on the surface. CD4 is a protein that binds to MHC class 2. Together this enables the helper T-cell to recognize antigens, and helps to activate helper T-cells.

The CD4 protein is also on the surface of monocytes, macrophages and dendritic cells.

CD8+ T-cells: These are cytotoxic T-cells that have CD8 on the surface. CD8 is a protein that binds to MHC class 1. Together this enables cell-signaling, which enables cytotoxic T-cells to recognize antigens, and helps to activate cytotoxic T-cells.

Cell-mediated immunity: Immunity that involves T-cells and their proliferation and activation, as well as the activation of phagocytes and cytokines, in response to the presence of antigens.

Chemokines: These are the dispatchers of the immune system. They induce chemotaxis, which is cell migration to where those cells are needed to fight infections.

Chemotaxis: Movement of a cell along a chemical concentration gradient, used by leukocytes to arrive to the location of infection.

Complement: Proteins in the innate especially and also the adaptive immune systems that directly destroy invaders or that signal pathogen presence to other cells in the immune system. They tag pathogens for phagocytosis.

Cytokines: Hormone-like messenger proteins, sent from one cell to another. Activated helper T-cells secrete cytokines that activate macrophages and B-cells, and can also promote inflammation.

Cytotoxic T-cells (CTL): Also called killer T-cells. These send toxic cytokines directly to infected cells, which kill the infected cells.

Dendritic cell (DC): A cell of the innate immune system that has many dendrites or limbs protruding that grab foreign proteins (antigens) in the tissues, then travel to lymphoid organs and display these antigens to T-cells, which activate the T-cells for adaptive immune response. See Antigen-presenting cells.

Helper T-cells (Th1 or Th2): These are activated by macrophages, in case of antigen invasion. The helper T-cells then secrete cytokines, specifically interleukins and interferons, in order to induce B-cells to produce antibodies to kill pathogens.

Hematopoiesis: The development and maturing of red and white blood cells in the bone marrow.

Humoral immunity: Immunity that involves B-cells and their proliferation and activation and antibody production, in response to the presence of antigens. This is the target of vaccines.

Immunoglobulins (Ig): Another name for antibodies, and a way to classify them: IgG is the most common and last longest. Others are IgM, IgA, IgE and IgD.

Inflammation: A surge of the immune system mostly involving macrophages and neutrophils as first responders to new invasive antigens.

Innate immune system: This is the older (in biological history) and more ubiquitous immune system throughout the body and throughout nature that all animal species are thought to have. (Only 1% have adaptive immunity). These are the first responders, the cells that inform and train the adaptive immune system in how to do battle against specific invading pathogens.

Interferons (IFN) alpha and beta: These are warning cytokines secreted by cells that have been infected by viruses. They interfere with viral replication.

Interferon (IFN) gamma: Natural killer cells and Th1 helper T-cells secrete this cytokine as activation for attack against antigens.

Interleukin (IL): Can be remembered by *inter:* between and *leuk* white blood cell. Interleukins are messenger communication molecules between white blood cells.

Killer T-cells: See Cytotoxic T-cells

Leukocytes: The soldiers of the immune system found in the blood stream. Also called white blood cells.

Lymph: Fluid that has leaked from blood into tissues, and carries waste products away from the tissues into the lymph system.

Lymphatic system: This is a one-way circulatory system in the body. It is a congregation site for the variety of cells in our immune system in their communication with each other. But it also picks up the cells killed in battle from both sides of conflict, excess mucous and similar debris from the immune system's war against invading pathogens. This debris-filled liquid is taken to the approximately 500 lymph nodes in the human body, and then to the lymphatic duct and the thoracic duct and the debris goes out with the stool, while the fluid is recycled to the circulatory system.

Lymphocytes: B-cells or T-cells.

Lysosome: A pocket at the membrane of our cells that is filled with acidic fluid and proteolytic (dissolving) enzymes that attack non-self intruders. Viruses use the acidic fluid to replicate.

Macrophages: From *macro-* (big) and *phage* (eater). Macrophages are generally the first of the first responders in the innate immune system. They are the most versatile cell in the immune system. They surround and engulf invading pathogens whole. Macrophages are also antigen-presenting cells, and can also kill invading pathogens directly.

Major histocompatibility complex (MHC) proteins: These are proteins that help with antigen presentation, mostly to T-cells. MHC-1 molecules are on the surface of most cells in the body, and display what is happening with viral activity inside the cells to cytotoxic T-cells, which kill infected cells. MHC-2 molecules are on antigen-presenting cells, such as macrophages. These signal to helper T-cells to secrete cytokines that induce B-cells to produce antibodies to kill pathogens.

Mast cells: Mast cells can kill pathogens directly. They release histamines and play a role in both innate and adaptive immunity, affecting the function of dendritic cells, T-cells, B-cells are other immune cells, as well as inflammatory responses.

Memory: To the immune system, memory involves recognizing the peculiarities of a previously invading pathogen. This is the role of the usually quiescent adaptive immune system on subsequent encounter with a known pathogen: Sudden, large-scale and efficient proliferation of T-cells and B-cells.

Microbes: Microscopic life forms, including bacteria, fungi, parasites and viruses. But viruses do not meet all agreed-on criteria for being alive.

Monocytes: A kind of white blood cells, which will later mature to be a macrophage or dendritic cell when and where this is needed.

Mucosa or mucous membranes: Surfaces that line the interior of the body, primarily in the respiratory and GI tracts.

Naïve lymphocytes: A B-cell or T-cell that has not yet been activated.

Natural killer cells (NK cells): Like neutrophils, natural killer cells stay in the bloodstream until recruited to sites of local infection, and exit the bloodstream to enter the tissue where needed. They are activated by Interferon-alpha or –beta from various other immune cells. Then they quickly proliferate, and secrete the cytokine Interferon-gamma, which with TNF, has effect in a positive feedback loop with macrophages to increase the numbers of NK cells and the activation of macrophages. NK cells kill bacteria, parasites, fungi and viruses.

Neutralizing antibody: An antibody that is successful in killing a pathogen or preventing a pathogen from entering or replicating in the cells that it aims to infect.

Neutrophils: A leukocyte that is short-lived and kamikaze deadly to invading pathogens. Normally speeding along its path in the bloodstream, when local macrophages emit the cytokine interleukin-1, the neutrophil gradually rolls to a stop in the bloodstream, sticks to the interior of the blood vessel wall, pries apart cells of the blood vessel walls, exits the bloodstream and goes into the tissues, where it is an active phagocyte.

Opsonized: A cell, such as a dendritic cell is opsonized or decorated on its surface with antigens or antibodies, in order to signal to or activate other immune system cells, such as T-cells.

Pathogen or Pathogenic microbe: The foreign invading microbe that has damaging potential in the body.

Peptide: A small part of a protein.

Phagocytes: From *phago-* (eating) and *cyte* (cell). These are cells that eat pathogens, surrounding and swallowing them whole usually. Macrophages and neutrophils engulf or phagocytose invading pathogens.

Plasma cells: Activated B-cells which produce a large amount of antibodies, then die.

Proliferation: Start making a lot of new cells of a particular type. Dangerous when cancer cells do it, but helpful with immune cells against an invading pathogen.

Receptors: Proteins on the surface of molecules that act as docking locations for incoming molecules. Usually those arriving molecules are helpful signals coming in from other cells in the body. But occasionally, they can be threatening, such as viruses. For example, in the case of SARS-CoV-2, the spike (or S) protein on the surface of the virus fits into the ACE2 receptor on our cells, which is a common and necessary receptor, very abundant in the lower respiratory tract. This is how SARS-CoV-2 arrives to create problems.

Regulatory T-cells: These inhibit the immune system from over-reacting to invading pathogens. We don't want such an overwhelming immune response that the tsunami of proliferating immune cells kills the patient. This is relevant to SARS-CoV-2. We see in the chapter on vitamin C and immune function that a deficiency of regulating T-cells allows SARS-CoV-2 to provoke overwhelming proliferation of excessive and ultimately suffocating neutrophils in the lungs.

T-cells Also called T-lymphocytes. The active agents in cell-mediated immunity. The larger part of the adaptive immune system, they last months to years. These are named T-cells, because they mature or differentiate in the thymus gland.

Th1 cells: A kind of CD4+ helper T-cell that secretes cytokines, including interferon-gamma, which stimulate phagocytes, such as macrophages and neutrophils.

Th2 cells: A kind of CD4+ helper T-cell that secretes cytokines such as IL-4, IL-5 and other cytokines that are involved in eosinophils' and mast cells' responses to allergenic antigens.

Thymus gland: A gland in the anterior mediastinum of the chest where T-cells mature.

Toll-like receptors: Receptors on the surface of cells that recognize and are alert to the presence of common invaders and generate warning signals for immune activation.

Tumor necrosis factor: A cytokine that can kill cancer cells and virus-infected cells, and can activate other immune system cells.

Virus: A parasitic entity that is arguably not alive because it is only a nucleic acid genome, DNA or RNA packaged inside of a protein capsid, inside a membrane envelope. However, it is arguably alive, because it acts in self-interest and replicates. But it cannot replicate on its own; it needs the cells of the host to do so.

White blood cells: See leukocytes.

References

Preface

[1] M Scholz, R Derwand, V Zelenko. COVID-19 outpatients – Early risk stratified treatment with zinc plus low dose hydroxychloroquine and azithromycin: A retrospective case series study. Dec 2020. Int J Antimicrob Agents. 56 (6). 106214. https://www.sciencedirect.com/science/article/pii/S0924857920304258

Introduction

[2] B Petrovska, S Cekovska. Extracts from the history and medical properties of garlic. Pharmacogn Rev. Jan-Jun 2010. 4 (7). 106-110. https://www.ncbi.nlm.nih.gov/pmc/articles/PMC3249897/

[3] J Paris. Pharmacologia, Corrected and extended, in accordance with the London Pharmacopoeia of 1824, and with the generally advanced state of chemical science, Volume 2. 1825. https://books.google.com/books?id=B5k-

AAAAYAAJ&printsec=frontcover&source=gbs_ge_summary_r&cad=0#v=onepage&q&f=false

[4] A Hopkins. The Scientific American Cyclopedia of Formulas: Partly Based Upon the 28th ed. Of Scientific American cyclopedia of receipts, notes and queries. Jun 26 2012. 878. https://books.google.com/books?id=ioNOAAAAMAAJ&lpg=PA878&ots=qeckOAeYsW&dq=marseilles%20vinegar&pg=PA878#v=onepage&q=marseilles%20vinegar&f=false

[5] S Percival. Aged garlic extract modifies human immunity. Feb 2016. J Nutr. 146 (2). 433S-436S. https://pubmed.ncbi.nlm.nih.gov/26764332/

[6] H Siddiqi, M Mehra. COVID-19 illness in native and immunosuppressed states: a clinical-therapeutic staging proposal. J Heart Lung Transplant. 39 (2020). 405-407. https://www.sciencedirect.com/science/article/pii/S105324982031473X

[7] J Rajter, M Sherman, et al. Use of ivermectin is associated with lower mortality in hospitalized patients with coronavirus disease 2019: The ivermectin in COVID nineteen study. Jan 2021. Chest. 159 (1). 85-92. https://www.sciencedirect.com/science/article/pii/S0012369220348984

[8] A Monette, A Mouland. T lymphocytes as measurable targets of protection and vaccination against viral disorders. Oct 24 2018. Int Rev Cell Mol Biol. https://www.ncbi.nlm.nih.gov/pmc/articles/PMC7104940/

[9] S Schmidt, G Pedersen, et al. Rational design and in vivo characterizations of vaccine adjuvants. Dec 31 2018. ILAR J. https://www.ncbi.nlm.nih.gov/pmc/articles/PMC6927902/

[10] M Aguado, J Barratt, et al. Report on WHO meeting on immunization in older adults: Geneva, Switzerland. Jan 12 2018. Vaccine. 36 (7). 921-931. https://www.ncbi.nlm.nih.gov/pmc/articles/PMC5865389/

[11] Y Zhou, Y Hou, et al. A network medicine approach to investigation and population-based validation of disease manifestations and drug repurposing for COVID-19. PLOS Biology. Nov 6 2020. https://journals.plos.org/plosbiology/article?id=10.1371/journal.pbio.3000970

[12] G Zhuang, M Shen, et al. Potential false-positive rate among the 'asymptomatic infected individuals' in close contacts of COVID-19 patients. https://www.researchgate.net/publication/339770271_Potential_false-positive_rate_among_the_'asymptomatic_infected_individuals'_in_close_contacts_of_COVID-19_patients

[13] US Health and Human Services, NVSS. Vital statistics reporting guidance. Apr 3, 2020. https://www.scribd.com/document/455607875/US-HHS-Document-to-Doctors-on-How-to-Certify-COVID-19-Deaths-including-Related-Deaths?campaign=VigLink&ad_group=xxc1xx&source=hp_affiliate&medium=affiliate

[14] M Rogers. Fact check: Hospitals get paid more if patients listed as COVID-19, on ventilators. USA Today. Apr 24, 2020. https://www.usatoday.com/story/news/factcheck/2020/04/24/fact-check-medicare-hospitals-paid-more-covid-19-patients-coronavirus/3000638001/

[15] K Waddill. Private payer COVID-19 reimbursement rates are twice Medicare rates. Health Payer Intelligence. Jul 13, 2020. https://healthpayerintelligence.com/news/private-payer-covid-19-reimbursement-rates-are-twice-medicare-rates

[16] American Hospital Association. Special Bulletin: Senate passes the Coronavirus Aid, Relief and Economic Security (CARES) Act. https://www.aha.org/special-bulletin/2020-03-26-senate-passes-coronavirus-aid-relief-and-economic-security-cares-act

[17] US Department of Health and Human Services. CARES Act Provider Relief Fund. HHS. https://www.hhs.gov/coronavirus/cares-act-provider-relief-fund/index.html

[18] M Rogers. Fact check: Hospitals get paid more if patients listed as COVID-19, on ventilators. USA Today. Apr 24 2020. https://www.usatoday.com/story/news/factcheck/2020/04/24/fact-check-medicare-hospitals-paid-more-covid-19-patients-coronavirus/3000638001/

[19] S Begley. With ventilators running out, doctors say the machines are overused for COVID-19. STAT. Apr 8 2020. https://www.statnews.com/2020/04/08/doctors-say-ventilators-overused-for-covid-19/

[20] K Mullis, interviewed. Every scary thing you're being told depends on the unreliable PCR test. English Rose. Bitchute video. https://www.bitchute.com/video/UbKDEvIG6m2t/

[21] US Centers for Disease Control and Prevention. Duration of isolation and precautions for adults with COVID-19. Oct 19 2020. https://www.cdc.gov/coronavirus/2019-ncov/hcp/duration-isolation.html

[22] M Landry. Your coronavirus test is positive. Maybe it shouldn't be. Clinical Virology Laboratory, Yale New Haven Hospital. https://medicine.yale.edu/labmed/sections/virology/COVID-19%20Ct%20values_YNHH%20Aug.%202020%20_395430_36854_v1.pdf

[23] A Mandavilli. Your coronavirus test is positive. Maybe it shouldn't be. New York Times. Aug 29 2020. https://www.nytimes.com/2020/08/29/health/coronavirus-testing.html

[24] Governor R DeSantis. Mandatory reporting of COVID-19 laboratory tests results: Reporting of cycle threshold values. Dec 3 2020. Florida Health. https://www.flhealthsource.gov/files/Laboratory-Reporting-CT-Values-12032020.pdf

[25] AACC. SARS-CoV-2 cycle threshold: a metric that matters (or not). Dec 3 2020. American Association for Clinical Chemistry. https://www.aacc.org/cln/cln-stat/2020/december/3/sars-cov-2-cycle-threshold-a-metric-that-matters-or-not

[26] J Bullard, K Dust, et al. Predicting infectious severe acute respiratory syndrome coronavirus 2 from diagnostic samples. Clin Infect Dis. 71 (10). Nov 15 2020. https://academic.oup.com/cid/article/71/10/2663/5842165

[27] J Strong, H Feldmann. The crux of Ebola diagnostics. J Infect Dis. Dec 1 2017 (216). https://academic.oup.com/jid/article/216/11/1340/4210467

[28] Technocracy News & Trends. Johns Hopkins: US death rate remains normal despite COVID-19. https://www.technocracy.news/johns-hopkins-u-s-death-rate-remains-normal-despite-covid-19/

[29] US Centers for Disease Control and Prevention. Daily updates of totals by week and state. Provisional death counts for coronavirus disease 2019 (COVID-19). National Center for Health Statistics. https://www.cdc.gov/nchs/nvss/vsrr/covid19/index.htm

[30] Event 201 https://youtu.be/AoLw-Q8X174

[31] US Centers for Disease Control and Prevention. Weekly updates by select demographic and geographic characteristics. Provisional death counts for coronavirus disease 2019 (COVID-19). National Center for Health Statistics. https://www.cdc.gov/nchs/nvss/vsrr/covid_weekly/

[32] BBC News. Covid death figures: 10 things we've learned. Oct 6 2020. https://www.bbc.com/news/uk-scotland-54433305

[33] H Salje, C Tran, et al. Estimating the burden of SARS-CoV-2 in France. Science. Jul 10 2020. https://science.sciencemag.org/content/369/6500/208

[34] J Ioannidis. Reconciling estimates of global spread and infection fatality rates of COVID-19: an overview of systematic evaluations. Mar 25 2021. Eur J Clin Inv. E13554. https://onlinelibrary.wiley.com/doi/pdfdirect/10.1111/eci.13554

[35] H Salje, C Tran, et al. Estimating the burden of SARS-CoV-2 in France. Science. Jul 10 2020. https://science.sciencemag.org/content/369/6500/208

[36] US Centers for Disease Control and Prevention. Deaths and mortality. National Center for Health Statistics. https://www.cdc.gov/nchs/fastats/deaths.htm

[37] J Goldstein, R Lee. Demographic perspectives on the mortality of COVID-19 and other epidemics. Proceedings of the National Academy of Sciences of the USA. Sep 8 2020. https://doi.org/10.1073/pnas.2006392117 https://www.pnas.org/content/117/36/22035#sec-3

[38] US Centers for Disease Control and Prevention. State and national provisional counts. National Vital Statistics System. https://www.cdc.gov/nchs/nvss/vsrr/provisional-tables.htm

[39] Revenue (sales) is reported for each company on Charles Schwab. https://www.schwab.com

[40] D deBara. 5 largest medical supply distributors. Biz2credit. May 27, 2020. https://www.biz2credit.com/blog/2020/05/27/5-largest-medical-supply-distributors/

[41] https://schwab.com

Air Products and Chemicals Inc **APD**:NYSE
Chemicals

Last Price	Today's Change	Bid/Size	Ask/Size	Today's Volume
$286.91	+0.66 (0.23%)	$280.09/1	$292.38/2	1,908,635 Above Avg.

As of close Friday, 01/15/2021

C **Schwab Equity Rating®** Data as of 01/08/2021*

First Quarter Earnings Announcement Expected

Trade
Margin Requirements

Summary | News | Charts | Ratings | **Earnings** | Statements | Peers | Ratios | Dividends | Reports | Options | Preferreds

Earnings | Estimates | Trends

Growth Analysis (Fiscal Year Ending September 30, 2020)

Vickers Insider Prophets Report | Reuters Investment Profile

Quarterly | Annual

Show Price Chart | Hide Price Chart

Earnings Per Share

Non-GAAP | **GAAP**

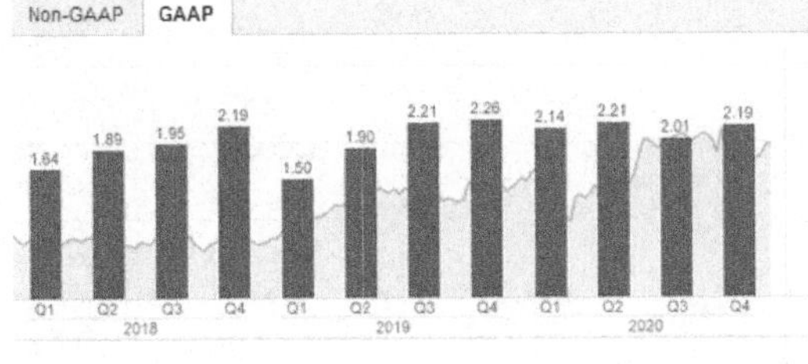

+14.8% **Annualized 5 Year growth rate**

Growth Rates (GAAP)

1 Yr	3 Yr	5 Yr
+8.5%	+18.3%	+14.8%

1 Yr Growth rate is trailing twelve months (TTM) compared to the previous twelve months. 3 and 5 Yr are compound annual growth rates (CAGR). Place your mouse over the bar to view GAAP and Non-GAAP results.

Positive/Negative Restatement | Recent Restatement

Revenue (Sales) (Numbers shown in Billions)

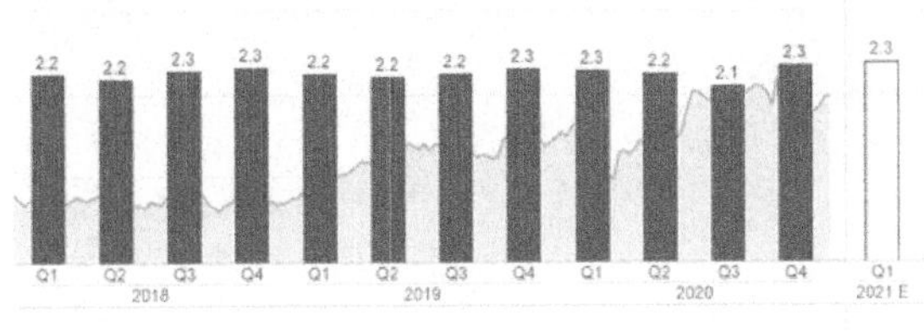

Current Quarter vs. Prior Year:

For the first quarter 2021, analysts estimate APD will generate revenues of $2.3B, an increase of 4.01% over the prior year first quarter results.

+2.5% **Annualized 5 Year growth rate**

Growth Rates

1 Yr	3 Yr	5 Yr
-0.7%	+2.7%	+2.5%

L'Air Liquide Societe Anonyme pour l'Etude et l'Exploitation des Procedes George **AIQUY** OTC Pink - Current Information OTC ADR

Chemicals

Last Price	Today's Change	ADR Ratio	Bid/Size	Ask/Size	Today's Volume
$32.89	**-0.18 (-0.54%)**	**5:1**	**$32.78**/1,000	**$33.64**/100	**90,191** Below Avg.

As of close Thursday, 12/31/2020

Schwab Equity Rating International® B within France, data as of 12/31/2020*

The Economist Intelligence Unit© BBB Country Risk Level as of 12/02/2020

You may be charged fees by the Bank that custodies this ADR. Read More about ADR pass-through fees.

This stock may be available for trading through a Schwab Global Account. Learn More

Trade

Compare Exchanges

Other Quotes For This Company

AIQUY OTC Pink - Curr...	**$USD 32.89**
AI:XPAR Euronext Paris	**€EUR 134.25**
AIQUF OTC Pink - Curr...	**$USD 167.06**

Quotes FAQ Margin Requirements

Summary News Charts Ratings Earnings **Statements** Peers Ratios Dividends Reports Options Preferreds

Income Statement Balance Sheet Cash Flow Statement

Income Statement (Fiscal Year Ending in December) *Converted Values in $USD*

Quarterly Annual

Detail View Summary View

Values are in Millions, except for per share data. Quarters are Fiscal Quarters. ( ) = Negative	Quarterly Trend	Q2 2020 6/30/2020 6 Months	Q4 2019 12/31/2019 6 Months	Q2 2019 6/30/2019 6 Months	Q4 2018 12/31/2018 6 Months	Q2 2018 6/30/2018 6 Months
Revenue & Gross Profit						
Total Revenue		***11,540***	***12,297***	***12,360***	***12,444***	***11,875***
Operating Expenses						
Cost of Revenue, Total		*4,079*	*4,399*	*4,774*	*4,964*	*4,614*
Labor & Related Expense		*2,452*	*2,497*	*2,464*	*2,414*	*2,386*
Sell/Gen/Admin Expenses, Total		*2,452*	*2,497*	*2,464*	*2,414*	*2,386*
Depreciation		*1,120*	*1,105*	*1,106*	*919*	*926*
Amortization of Intangibles		*98*	*99*	*94*	*99*	*101*

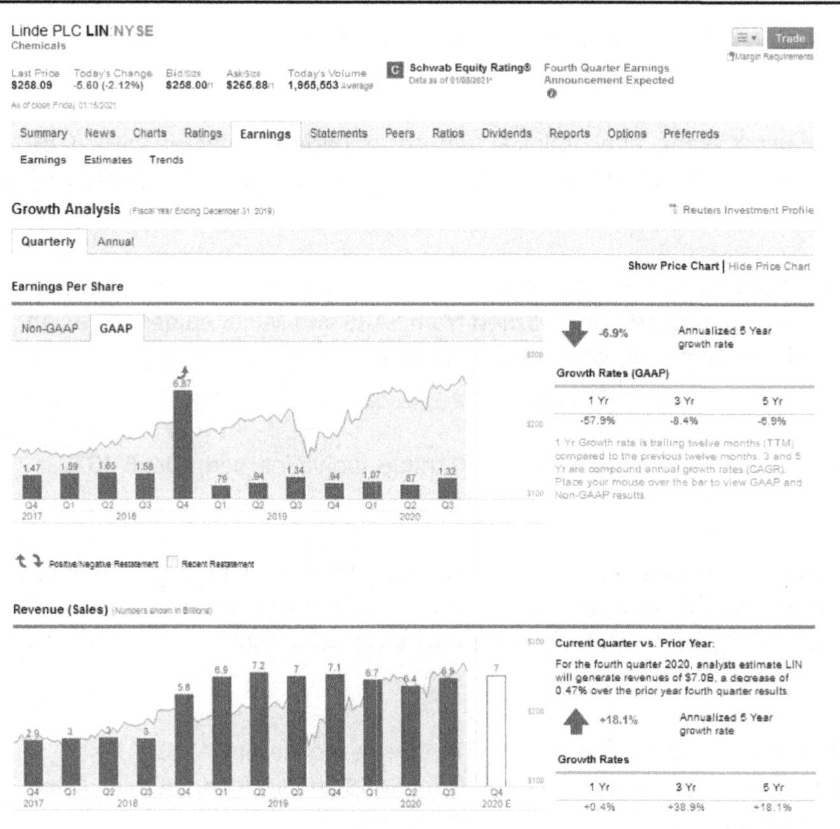

Part II

[42] A Patri, G Fabbrocini. Hydroxychloroquine and ivermectin: a synergistic combination for COVID-19 chemoprophylaxis and/or treatment? Jun 2020. J Am Acad Dermatol. 82 (6). https://www.ncbi.nlm.nih.gov/pmc/articles/PMC7146719/

[43] C Huang, Y Wang, et al. Clinical features of patients infected with 2019 novel coronavirus in Wuhan, China. Lancet. Feb 15 2020. 395 (10223): 497-506. https://pubmed.ncbi.nlm.nih.gov/31986264/

[44] E Prompetchara, C Ketloy, et al. Immune responses in COVID-19 and potential vaccines: Lessons learned from SARS and MERS epidemic. Asian Pac J Allergy Immunol. Mar 2020. 38 (1). 1-9. https://pubmed.ncbi.nlm.nih.gov/32105090/

[45] BBC News. Covid death figures: 10 things we've learned. Oct 6 2020. https://pubmed.ncbi.nlm.nih.gov/25903964/

[46] J Downing, H Martinez-Valdez, et al. Hyperthermia in humans enhances interferon-gamma synthesis and alters the peripheral lymphocyte population. J Interferon Res. Apr 1988. 8 (2). 143-150. https://pubmed.ncbi.nlm.nih.gov/3132509/

[47] E Prompetchara, C Ketloy, et al. Immune responses in COVID-19 and potential vaccines: Lessons learned from SARS and MERS epidemic. Asian Pac J Allergy Immunol. Mar 2020. 38 (1). 1-9. https://pubmed.ncbi.nlm.nih.gov/32105090/

[48] J Hadjadj, N Yatim, et al. Impaired Type I interferon activity and inflammatory responses in severe COVID-19 patients. Science. Aug 7 2020. 369 (6504). 718-724. https://pubmed.ncbi.nlm.nih.gov/32661059/

[49] P Bastard, L Rosen, et al. Autoantibodies against type I IFNs in patients with life threatening COVID-19. Science. Oct 23 2020. 370 (6515). eabd4585. https://pubmed.ncbi.nlm.nih.gov/32972996/

[50] E Ernst, E Pecho, et al. Regular sauna bathing and the incidence of common colds. Ann Med. 1990. 22 (4). 225-227. https://pubmed.ncbi.nlm.nih.gov/2248758/

[51] P Lang, N Samaras, et al. How important is vitamin D in preventing infections? Nov 17 2012. Ostep Intl. 24. 1537-1553. https://link.springer.com/article/10.1007/s00198-012-2204-6

[52] M Cantorna Vitamin D and autoimmunity: is vitamin D status an environmental factor affecting autoimmune disease prevalence? Proc Soc Exp Biol Med. Mar 2000. 223 (3). 230-233. https://pubmed.ncbi.nlm.nih.gov/10719834/

[53] H DeLuca, M Cantorna. Vitamin D: its role and uses in immunology. FASEB J. Dec 1 2001. 15(14. 2579-2585. https://faseb.onlinelibrary.wiley.com/doi/full/10.1096/fj.01-0433rev

[54] M Cantorna, C Munsick, et al. 1,25-dihyroxycholecalciferol prevents and ameliorates symptoms of experimental murine inflammatory bowel disease. J Nutr. Nov 2000. 130 (11). 2648-52. https://pubmed.ncbi.nlm.nih.gov/11053501/

[55] J Zella and H DeLuca. Vitamin D status and autoimmune diabetes in NOD/Ltj mice. FASEB J. J Cell Biochem. Feb 1 2003. 88 (2). 216-222. https://pubmed.ncbi.nlm.nih.gov/12520517/

[56] M Cantorna, C Hayes, et al. 1,25-dihydroxycholecalciferol inhibits the progression of arthritis in murine models of human arthritis. J Nutr. Jan 1998. 128 (1). 68-72. J Nutr. Jan 1998. 128 (1). 68-72. https://pubmed.ncbi.nlm.nih.gov/9430604/

[57] D D'Ambrosio, M Cippitelli, et al. Inhibition of IL-12 production by 1,25 dyhydroxyvitamin D3. Involvement of NF-kappa-B downregulation in transcriptional repression of the p40 gene. J Clin Invest Dec 31 1997. 101 (1). 252-262. https://europepmc.org/article/PMC/508562

[58] X Dong, T Craig, et al. Direct transcriptional regulation of RelB by 1 alsopha, 25-dihydroxyvitamin D3 and its analogs: physiologic and therapeutic implications for dendritic cell function. J Biol Chem. Sep 23 2003. 278 (49). 49378-49385. https://europepmc.org/article/MED/14507914

[59] X Dong, W Lutz, et al. Regulation of relB in dendritic cells by means of modulated association of vitamin D receptor and histone deascetylase 3 with the promoter. Proc Natl Acad Sci. Nov 1 2005. 102 (44). 16007-16012. https://europepmc.org/article/MED/16239345#abstract

[61] S Hansdottir, M Monick, et al. Vitamin D decreases respiratory syncytial virus induction of NF-kappa-B,linked chemokines and cytokines in airway epithelium while maintaining the antiviral state. J Immunol. Dec 10 2009. 184 (2). 965-974. https://europepmc.org/article/PMC/3035054

[62] J LeMire, D Archer, et al. Prolongation of the survival of murine cardiac allografts by the Vitamin D3 analogue 1,25-dihydroxy-L16-cholecalciferol. Transplantation. Oct 1992. 54 (4). 762-763. https://pubmed.ncbi.nlm.nih.gov/1412777/

[63] L McLaughlin, L Clarke, et al. Vitamin D for the treatment of multiple sclerosis: a meta-analysis. Neurol. Dec 2018. 265 (12). 2893-2905. https://pubmed.ncbi.nlm.nih.gov/30284038/

[64] J Matías-Guíu, C Oreja-Guevara, et al. Vitamin D and remyelination in multiple sclerosis. Neurología. Apr 2018. 33 (3). 177-186. https://pubmed.ncbi.nlm.nih.gov/27321170/

[65] M Cantorna, C Hayes, et al. 1,25-dihydroxyvitamin D3 reversibly blocks the progression of relapsing encephalomyelitis, a model of multiple sclerosis. Pro Natl Acad Sci. Jul 23 1996. 93 (15). 7861-4 https://pubmed.ncbi.nlm.nih.gov/8755567/

[66] A Martineau, D Joliffe, et al. Vitamin D supplementation to prevent acute respiratory tract infections: systematic review and meta-analysis of individual participant data. BMJ. Feb 15 2017. 356:i6583. https://pubmed.ncbi.nlm.nih.gov/28202713/

[67] S Esposito, M Lelii. Vitamin D and respiratory tract infections in childhood. BMC Infect Dis. 2015. 15:487. https://bmcinfectdis.biomedcentral.com/track/pdf/10.1186/s12879-015-1196-1.pdf

[68] H Brenner, B Holleczek, et al. Vitamin D insufficiency and deficiency and mortality from respiratory diseases in a cohort of older adults: potential for limiting the death toll during and beyond the COVID-19 pandemic? Nutrients. Aug 18 2020. 12 (8): 2488. https://pubmed.ncbi.nlm.nih.gov/32824839/

[69] O Gutiérrez, W Farwell, et al. Racial differences in the relationship between vitamin D, bone mineral density, and parathyroid hormone in the National Health and Nutrition Examination Survey. Osteop Intl. 2011. 22. 1745-1753. https://link.springer.com/article/10.1007/s00198-010-1383-2

[70] J MacLaughlin, MF Holick. Aging decreases the capacity of human skin to produce vitamin D3. J Clin Invest. Oct 1985. 76 (4): 1536-8. https://pubmed.ncbi.nlm.nih.gov/2997282/

[71] J Wortsman, L Matsuoka, et al. Decreased bioavailability of vitamin D in obesity. Am J Clin Nutr. 72 (3). Sep 2000. 690-693. https://academic.oup.com/ajcn/article/72/3/690/4729361

[72] N Klepeis, W Nelson, et al. The National Human Activity Pattern Survey (NHAPS): a resource for assessing exposure to environmental pollutants. J Expo Anal Environ Epidemiol. May-Jun 2001. 11 (3): 231-252. https://pubmed.ncbi.nlm.nih.gov/11477521/

[73] C Huber. Masks, false safety and real dangers. Proposed mechanisms by which masks increase risk of COVID-19. PDMJ. Jan 8 2021. https://pdmj.org/papers/masks_false_safety_and_real_dangers_part4/

[74] P Liu, S Stenger, et al. Toll-like receptor triggering of a vitamin D-mediated human antimicrobial response. Science. Feb 22 2006. 311 (5768). 1770-1773. https://europepmc.org/article/MED/16497887

[75] P Barlow, P Svoboda, et al. Antiviral activity and increased host defense against influenza infection elicited by the human cathelicidin LL-37. PLoS One. Oct 20 2011. https://europepmc.org/article/PMC/3198734

[76] C Gunville, P Mourani, et al. The role of vitamin D in prevention and treatment of infection. Infl & Allergy Drug Targets. Jul 31 2013. 12 (4). 239-245. https://europepmc.org/article/PMC/3756814#R6

[77] S Iacob, E Panaitescu, et al. The human cathelicidin LL37 peptide has high plasma levels in B and C hepatitis related to viral activity but not to 25-hydroxyvitamin D plasma level. Rom J Intern Med. Jun 30 2012. 50 (3). 217-223. https://europepmc.org/article/MED/23330289

[78] B Ramanathan, E Davis, et al. Cathelicidins: microbicidal activity, mechanisms of action, and roles in innate immunity. Microbes Infect. 2002. 4 (3). 361-372. . https://europepmc.org/article/MED/11909747

[79] J White. Vitamin D as inducer of cathelicidin antimicrobial peptide expression: past, present and future. J Steroid Biochem Mol Biol. 2010. 121 (1-2). 234 – 238. Mar 16 2010. 121 (1-2). 234 – 238. https://europepmc.org/article/MED/20302931

[80] S Yim, P Dhawan, et al. IOnduction of cathelicidin in normal and CF brochial epithelial cells by 1,25-dihydroxyvitamin D3. Cyst Fibros. Apr 26 2007. 6 (6). 403-410. https://europepmc.org/article/PMC/2099696

[81] B Ramanathan, E Davis, et al. Cathelicidins: microbiocidal activity, mechanisms of action, and roles in innate immunity. Microbes Infect. Feb 28 2002. 4 (3). 361-372. https://europepmc.org/article/MED/11909747

[82] A Van der Does, P Bergman, et al. Induction of the human cathelicidin LL-37 as a novel treatment against bacterial infections. J Leukoc Biol. Jun 12 2012. 92 (4). 735-742. https://europepmc.org/article/MED/22701042

[83] P Liu, S Stenger, et al. Toll-like receptor triggering of a vitamin D-mediated human antimicrobial response. Science. Mar 24 2006. 311 (5768): 1770-3. https://pubmed.ncbi.nlm.nih.gov/16497887/

[84] R Chun, P Liu, et al. Impact of vitamin D on immune function: lessons learned from genome-wide analysis. Front. Physiol. Apr 21 2014. 5 (151). https://pubmed.ncbi.nlm.nih.gov/24795646/

[85] E Abe, C Miyaura, et al. Differentiation of mouse myeloid leukemia cells induced by a 1alpha,25-dihydroxybitamin D3. Proc Natl Acad Sci. Aug 1981. 4990-4994. https://pubmed.ncbi.nlm.nih.gov/6946446/

[86] H Tanaka, E Abe, et al. 1alpha, 25 di-hydroxycholecalciferol and a human myeloid leukaemia cell line (HL-60). The presence of a cytosol receptor and induction of differentiation. Biochem J. Jun 1982. 204 (3). 713-719. https://pubmed.ncbi.nlm.nih.gov/6289803/

[87] Y Abu-Amer, Z Bar-Shavit. Impaired bone marrow-derived macrophage differentiation in vitamin D deficiency. Cell Immunol. Oct 15 1993. 151 (2). 356-368. https://pubmed.ncbi.nlm.nih.gov/8402942/

[88] G Bomfim, L Overbergh, et al. 1a,25-dihydroxyvitamin D3 and its analogs as modulators of human dendritic cells: a comparison dose-titration study. J Steroid Biochem Mol Biol. Jul 2013. 136: 160-165. https://pubmed.ncbi.nlm.nih.gov/23098690/

[89] E van Etten, C Mathieu. Immunoregulation by 1,25-dihydroxyvitamin D3: basic concepts. J Steroid Biochem Mol Biol. Oct 2005. 97 (1-2). 93-101. https://pubmed.ncbi.nlm.nih.gov/16046118/

[90] J Mora, M Iwata, et al. Vitamin effects on the immune system: vitamins A and D take centre stage. Nat Rev Immunol. 2008. 8 (9). 685-698. Nature Reviews. Immunol. Aug 31 2008. 8 (9). 685-698. https://europepmc.org/article/PMC/2906676

[91] S Hansdottir, M Monick, et al. Respiratory epithelial cells convert inactive vitamin D to its active form: potential effects on host defense. J Immunol. Oct 31 2008. 181 (10). 7090-7099. 181 (10). 7090-7099. https://europepmc.org/article/PMC/2596683

Vitamin D in the adaptive immune system

[92] B Bridle. Coronavirus vaccine concerns: "I would prefer to have natural immunity." Feb 24 2021. Dryburgh.com. https://dryburgh.com/byram-bridle-coronavirus-vaccine-concerns/

[93] S Manolagas, D Provvedini, et al. Interactions of 1,25-dihydroxyvitamin D3 and the immune system. Mol Cell Endocrinol. Dec 1985. 43 (2-3). 113-22. https://pubmed.ncbi.nlm.nih.gov/3000847/

[94] X Yu, H Mocharla, et al. Vitamin D receptor expression in human lymphocytes. Signal requirements and characterization by western blots and DNA sequencing. Apr 25 1991. J Biol Chem. 266 (12). 7588-95. https://pubmed.ncbi.nlm.nih.gov/1850412/

[95] R Wiese, A Uhland-Smith, et al. Up-regulation of the vitamin D receptor in response to 1,25-dihydroxyvitamin D3 results from ligand-induced stabilization. J Biol Chem. 267. 20082-20086. https://pubmed.ncbi.nlm.nih.gov/1328192/

[96] M Cantorna. Mechanisms underlying the effect of vitamin D on the immune system. Cambridge Univ Press. Jun 2 2010. https://www.cambridge.org/core/journals/proceedings-of-the-nutrition-society/article/mechanisms-underlying-the-effect-of-vitamin-d-on-the-immune-system/91FB1F56494E909053590AE99E4C6DC4

[97] J Lemire, D Archer, et al. Immmunosuppressive actions of 1,25-dihydroxyvitamin D3: preferential inhibition of TH1 functions. J Nutr Jun 1995. 125 (6 Suppl). 1704S-1708S. https://academic.oup.com/jn/article-abstract/125/suppl_6/1704S/4730957?redirectedFrom=fulltext

[98] I Alroy, T Towers, et al. Transcriptional repression of the interleukin-2 gene by vitamin D3: Direct inhibition of NFAT//AP-1 complex formation by a nuclear hormone receptor. Oct 1 1995. Am Soc Microbio J https://mcb.asm.org/content/15/10/5789

---

[99] J Adams, M Hewison. Unexpected actions of vitamin D: new perspectives on the regulation of innate and adaptive immunity. Nat Clin Pract Endocrinol Metab. Jan 31 2008. 4 (2). 80-90. https://europepmc.org/article/PMC/2678245

[100] M Hewison. An update on vitamin D and human immunity. Clin Endocrinol (Oxf). Feb 29 2012. 76 (3). 315-325. https://europepmc.org/article/MED/21995874

[101] F Baeke, H Korf, et al. The vitamin D analog TX527, promotes a human CD4, CD25high, CD127 low regulatory T cell profile and induces a migratory signature specific for homing to sites of inflammation. Jan 1 2011. J Immunol. 186 (1). 132-142. https://www.jimmunol.org/content/186/1/132.long

[102] M Kongsbak, T Levring, et al. The vitamin D receptor and T cell function. Jun 18 2013. Front Immunol. https://www.frontiersin.org/articles/10.3389/fimmu.2013.00148/full#B8

[103] Hansdottir, M Monick, et al. Respiratory epithelial cells convert inactive vitamin D to its active form: potential effects on host defense. J Immunol. Oct 31 2008. 181 (10). 7090 – 7099. https://europepmc.org/article/PMC/2596683

[104] P Smith, G Lombardi, et al. Type I interferons and the innate immune response-more than just antiviral cytokines. Mol Immunol. Jan 12 2005. 42 (8). 869-877. https://europepmc.org/article/MED/15829276

[105] J Hiscott. Triggering the innate antiviral response through IRF-3 activation. J Biol Chem. Mar 28 2007. 282 (21). 15325-15329. https://europepmc.org/article/MED/17395583

[106] A Stoppelenburg, J von Hegedus, et al. Defective control of vitamin D receptor-mediated epithelial STAT1 signalling predisposes to severe respiratory syncytial virus bronchiolitis. J Path. 232 (1). 57-64. https://onlinelibrary.wiley.com/doi/abs/10.1002/path.4267

[107] A Hornsleth, L Loland, et al. Cytokines and chemokines in respiratory secretion and severity of disease in infants with respiratory syncytial virus (RSV) infection. Apr 30 2001. 21 (2). 163-170. https://europepmc.org/article/MED/11378497

[108] J Van Woensel and J Kimpen. Therapy for respiratory tract infections caused by respiratory syncytial virus. Eur J Ped. May 31 2000. 159 (6). 391-398. https://europepmc.org/article/MED/10867842

[109] S Hansdottir, M Monick, et al. Vitamin D decreases respiratory syncytial virus induction of NF-kappa-B-linked chemokines and cytokines in airway epithelium while maintaining the antiviral state. J Immunol. Dec 10 2009. 184 (2). 965-974. https://europepmc.org/article/PMC/3035054#R80

[110] E Villamor. A potential role for vitamin D on HIV infection? Nutr Rev. 64 (5). May 2006. 226-233. https://academic.oup.com/nutritionreviews/article/64/5/226/1910640

[111] R Connor, W Rigby. 1 alpha, 25-dihydroxyvitamin D3 inhibits productive infection of human monocytes by HIV-1 Biochem Biophys Res Comm. Mar 31 1991. 176 (2). 852-859. https://www.sciencedirect.com/science/article/abs/pii/S0006291X05802645?via%3Dihub

[112] A Braun, D Chang, et al. Association of low serum 25-hydroxyvitamin D levels and mortality in the critically ill. Crit Care Med. Mar 31 2011. 39 (4). 671-677. https://europepmc.org/article/PMC/3448785

[113] L Mathews, Y Ahmed, et al. Worsening severity of vitamin D deficiency is associated with increased length of stay, surgical intensive care unit cost, and mortality rate in surgical intensive care unit patients. Am J Surg. Feb 9 2012. 204 (1). 37-43. https://europepmc.org/article/PMC/3992708

[114] A Ginde, J Mansbach, et al. Association between serum 25-hydroxyvitamin D level and upper respiratory tract infection in the Third National health and Nutrition Examination Survey. Arch Intern Med. Jan 31 2009. 169 (4). 384-390. https://europepmc.org/article/PMC/3447082

[115] L Leow, T Simpson, et al. Vitamin D, innate immunity and outcomes in community acquired pneumonia. Respirology. Apr 30 2011. 16 (4). 611-616. https://onlinelibrary.wiley.com/doi/full/10.1111/j.1440-1843.2011.01924.x

[116] L Muhe, S Lulseged, et al. Case-control study of the role of nutritional rickets in the risk of developing pneumonia in Ethiopian children. Lancet. May 31 1997. 349 (9068). 1801-1804. https://europepmc.org/article/MED/9269215

[117] V Wayse, A Yousafzai, et al. Association of subclinical vitamin D deficiency with severe acute lower respiratory infection in Indian children under 5 years. Eur J Clin Nutr. Mar 31 2004. 58 (4). 563-567. https://www.nature.com/articles/1601845

[118] J McNally, K Menon, et al. The association of vitamin D status with pediatric critical illness. Pediatrics. Aug 5 2012. 130 (3). 429-436. https://europepmc.org/article/MED/22869837

Vitamin D vs COVID

[119] J Ioannidis. Infection fatality rate of COVID-19 inferred from seroprevalence data. World Health Organization. May 13 2020. https://www.who.int/bulletin/volumes/99/1/20-265892/en/

[120] J Ioannidis. Reconciling estimates of global spread and infection fatality rates of COVID-19: an overview of systematic evaluation. Mar 26 2021. Eur J Clin Inv. https://onlinelibrary.wiley.com/doi/10.1111/eci.13554

[121] W Grant, H Lahore, et al. Evidence that vitamin D supplementation could reduce risk of influenza and COVID-19 infections and deaths. Nutr Mar 12 2020. 12 (4). 988. https://www.mdpi.com/2072-6643/12/4/988.

[122] L Chen, X Yang, et al. Dysregulated renin-angiotensis system contributes to acute lung injury caused by hind-limb ischemia-reperfusion in mice. Nov 2013. 40 (5). 420-429. https://journals.lww.com/shockjournal/Fulltext/2013/11000/Dysregulated_Renin_AngioteNsin_System_Contributes.12.aspx

[123] R Mardani, A Alamdary, et al. Association of vitamin D with the modulation of the disease severity in COVID-19. Virus Res. Nov 2020. 289 (198148). https://www.ncbi.nlm.nih.gov/pmc/articles/PMC7455115/

[124] E Williamson, A Walker, et al. Factors associated with COVID-19-related death using OpenSAFELY. Nature. Aug 2020. 584 (7821). 430-436. https://pubmed.ncbi.nlm.nih.gov/32640463/

[125] CDC. Body mass index and risk for COVID-19-related hospitalization, intensive care unit admission, invasive mechanical ventilation, and death – United States, March-December 2020. Mar 12 2021. MMWR. 70 (10). 355-361. https://www.cdc.gov/mmwr/volumes/70/wr/mm7010e4.htm?s_cid=mm7010e4_w

[126] J Rhodes, S Subramanian, et al. Editorial: low population mortality from COVID-19 in countries south of latitude 35 degrees North support vitamin D as a factor determining severity. Aliment Pharmacol Ther. Jun 2020. 51 (12). 1434-1437. https://pubmed.ncbi.nlm.nih.gov/32311755/

[127] P Ilie, S Stefanescu, et al. The role of vitamin D in the prevention of coronavirus disease 2019 infection and mortality. Aging Clin Exp Res. Mar 30 2020. https://www.ncbi.nlm.nih.gov/pmc/articles/PMC7202265/pdf/40520_2020_Article_1570.pdf

[128] A D'Avolio, V Avataneo, et al. 25-hydroxyvitamin D concentrations are lower in patients with positive PCR for SARS-CoV-2. Nutrients. Apr 20 2020. 12 (5). https://www.mdpi.com/2072-6643/12/5/1359

[129] M Demir, F Demir, et al. Vitamin D deficiency is associated with COVID-19 positivity and severity of the disease. J Med Vir. Jan 29 2021. https://onlinelibrary.wiley.com/doi/10.1002/jmv.26832

[130] A Abdollahi, H Sarvestani, et al. The association between the level of serum 25(OH) vitamin D, obesity and underlying diseases with the risk of developing COVID-19 infection: A case-control study of hospitalized patients in Tehran, Iran. J Med Virol. Dec 12 2020. https://onlinelibrary.wiley.com/doi/10.1002/jmv.26726

[131] A Faniyi, S Lugg, et al. Vitamin D status and seroconversion for COVID-19 in UK healthcare workers. Eur. Respir J 2020. https://erj.ersjournals.com/content/erj/early/2020/11/26/13993003.04234-2020.full.pdf

[132] E Merzon, D Tworowski, et al. Low plasma 25 (OH) vitamin D level is associated with increased risk of COVID-19 infection: an Israeli population-based study. FEBS J Sep 2020. 287 (17): 3693-3702. https://pubmed.ncbi.nlm.nih.gov/32700398/

[133] A Radukovic, A Hippchen, et al. Vitamin D deficiency and outcome of COVID-19 patients. Nutrients Sep 1 2020. 12 (9). 2757. https://www.mdpi.com/2072-6643/12/9/2757/htm

[134] H Kaufman, J Niles. SARS-CoV-2 positivity rates associated with circulating 25-hydroxyvitamin D levels. PLoS One. Sep 17 2020. 15 (9). E00239252. https://pubmed.ncbi.nlm.nih.gov/32941512/

[135] A Jain, R Chaurasia, et al. Analysis of vitamin D level among asymptomatic and critically ill COVID-19 patients and its correlation with inflammatory markers. Sci Rep. Nov 19 2020. 10 (1) 20191. https://pubmed.ncbi.nlm.nih.gov/33214648/

[136] A Radujkovic, T Hippchen. Vitamin D deficiency and outcome of COVID-19 patients. Nutrients. Aug 9 2020. 12 (9). 2757. https://www.mdpi.com/2072-6643/12/9/2757/htm

[137] H Susianti, C Wahono, et al. Low levels of vitamin D were associated with coagulopathy among hospitalized coronavirus (COVID-19) patients: a single-centered study in Indonesia. J Med Biochem Feb 12 2021. https://aseestant.ceon.rs/index.php/jomb/article/view/30228

[138] M Infante, A Buoso, et al. Low vitamin D status at admission as a risk factor for poor survival in hospitalized patients with COVID-19: An Italian retrospective study. J Am Coll Nutrition. Oct 31 2020. https://www.tandfonline.com/doi/full/10.1080/07315724.2021.1877580

[139] P Vanegas-Cedillo, O Bello-Chavolla, et al. Serum vitamin D levels are associated with increased COVID severity and mortality independent of visceral adiposity. Mar 14 2020. MedRxiv. https://www.medrxiv.org/content/10.1101/2021.03.12.21253490v2

[140] S Ling, E Broad, et al. High-dose cholecalciferol booster therapy is associated with a reduced risk of mortality in patients with COVID-19: A cross-sectional multi-centre observational study. Nov 15 2020. Nutrients. 12 (12). 3799. https://www.mdpi.com/2072-6643/12/12/3799/htm

[141] N Charroenngam, A Shirvani, et al. Association of vitamin D status with hospital morbidity and mortality in adult hospitalized COVID-19 patients. Mar 8 2021. Endo Practice. https://www.endocrinepractice.org/article/S1530-891X(21)00057-4/fulltext

[142] A Ahmad, C Heumann, et al. Mean vitamin D levels in 19 European countries & COVID-19 mortality over 10 months. Mar 12 2021. MedRxiv. https://www.medrxiv.org/content/10.1101/2021.03.11.21253361v1

[143] S Walrand. Autumn COVID-19 surge dates in Europe correlated to latitudes, not to temperature-humidity, pointing to vitamin D as contributing factor. Jan 21 2021. Sci Rep. 11 (1981). https://www.nature.com/articles/s41598-021-81419-w

[144] J Cannell, R Vieth, et al. Epidemic influenza and vitamin D. Sep 7 2006. Epidem Inf. 134 (6). 1129-1140. https://www.cambridge.org/core/journals/epidemiology-and-infection/article/epidemic-influenza-and-vitamin-d/C4D90C6E7CB127E6DF7A52D3A9EE2974

[145] L Pedersen, F Nashold, et al. 1,25-dihydroxyvitamin D3 reverses experimental autoimmune encephalomyelitis by inhibiting chemokine synthesis and monocyte trafficking. J Neurosci Res. 85 (11). 2480-2490. https://europepmc.org/article/MED/17600374

[146] N Giarratana, G Penna, et al. A vitamin D analog down-regulates proinflammatory chemokine production by pancreatic islets inhibiting T cell recruitment and type 1 diabetes development. J Immunol. Jul 31 2004. 173 (4). 2280-2287. https://europepmc.org/article/MED/15294940

[147] C Gysemans, A Cardozo, et al. 1,25-dihydroxyvitamin D3 modulates expression of chemokines and cytokines in pancreatic islets: implications for prevention of diabetes in nonobese diabetic mice. Endocrin. Jan 5 2005. 146 (4). 1956-1964. https://europepmc.org/article/MED/15637289

[148] C Huber. COVID-19 is a lack of nutrients, exploited by a virus. PrimaryDoctor. Aug 28 2020. https://www.primarydoctor.org/covid-19-is-a-lack-of-nutrients

[149] R Dancer, D Parekh, et al. Vitamin D deficiency contributes directly to the acute respiratory distress syndrome. Thorax. Jul 2015. 70 (7). 617-624. https://pubmed.ncbi.nlm.nih.gov/25903964/

[150] A Sulli, E Gotelli, et al. Vitamin D and lung outcomes in elderly COVID-19 patients. Nutrients. 13 (3) Jan 2021. https://www.mdpi.com/2072-6643/13/3/717

[151] G Mazziotti, E Lavezzi, et al. Vitamin D deficiency, secondary hyperparathyroidism and respiratory insufficiency in hospitalized patients with COVID-19. J Endo Inves. Mar 5 2021. https://link.springer.com/article/10.1007/s40618-021-01535-2

[152] K Cashman, K Dowling, et al. Vitamin D deficiency in Europe: Pandemic? Am J Clin Nutr Feb 10 2016. 103 (4). 1033-1044. https://academic.oup.com/ajcn/article/103/4/1033/4662891

[153] T Griffin, D Wall, et al. Vitamin D status of adults in the community, in outpatient clinics, in hospital, and in nursing homes in the west of Ireland. J Gerontol. 75 (12). Dec 2020. 2418-2425. https://academic.oup.com/biomedgerontology/article-abstract/75/12/2418/5703038?redirectedFrom=fulltext

[154] T Clemens, J Adams, et al. Measurement of circulating vitamin D in man. Clin Chim Acta. Jun 3 1982. 121 (3). 301-308. https://pubmed.ncbi.nlm.nih.gov/6286167/

[155] I Murai, A Fernandes, et al. Effect of a single high dose of vitamin D3 on hospital length of stay in patients with moderate to severe COVID-19: A randomized clinical trial. JAMA. Feb 17 2021. e2026848. https://pubmed.ncbi.nlm.nih.gov/33595634/

[156] M Entrenas L Entrenas, et al. Effect of calcifediol treatment and best available therapy versus best available therapy on intensive care unit admission and mortality among patients hospitalized for COVID-19: A pilot randomized clinical study. J Steroid Biochem Mol Biol. Oct 2020. 203:105751. https://pubmed.ncbi.nlm.nih.gov/32871238/

[157] M Lakireddy, S Gadiga, et al. Impact of pulse D therapy on the inflammatory markers in patients with COVID-19. Research Square. Feb 23 2021. https://www.researchsquare.com/article/rs-152494/v1

[158] D Murdoch, S Slow et al. Effect of vitamin D3 supplementation on upper respiratory tract infections in healthy adults: the Vidaris randomized controlled trial. JAMA. Sep 30 2012. 308 (13). 1333-1339. https://europepmc.org/article/MED/23032549

[159] M Urashima, T Segawa, et al. Randmized trial of vitamin D supplementation to prevent seasonal influenza A in schoolchildren. Am J Clin Nutr. Mar 9 2010. 91 (5). 1255-1260. https://europepmc.org/article/MED/20219962

[160] J Charan, J Goyal, et al. Vitamin D for prevention of respiratory tract infections: A systematic review and meta-analysis. J Pharmacol & Pharmacotherapeutics. Sep 30 2012. 3 (4). 300-303. https://europepmc.org/article/PMC/3543548

[161] H Bischoff-Ferrari, W Willett, et al. Fracture prevention with vitamin D supplementation. JAMA. May 11 2005. https://jamanetwork.com/journals/jama/article-abstract/200871

[162] C Huber. Defeating cancer requires more than one treatment method: An 11-year retrospective case series using multiple nutritional and herbal agents, 2017 update. Dec 30 2017. https://natureworksbest.com/wp-content/uploads/2018/01/2017-Cancer-treatment-paper.2017.12.30.pdf

[163] J Ekwaru, J Zwicker, et al. The importance of body weight for the dose response relationship of oral vitamin D supplementation and serum 25-hydroxyvitamin D in healthy volunteers. PLoS One. Nov 5 2014. https://journals.plos.org/plosone/article?id=10.1371/journal.pone.0111265

[164] C Jacobus, M Holick, et al. Hypervitaminosis D associated with drinking milk. NEJM. Apr 30 1992. 326: 1173-1177. https://www.nejm.org/doi/full/10.1056/NEJM199204303261801

[165] IOM (Institute of Medicine) Dietary Reference Intakes for Calcium and Vitamin D. Washington, DC: National Academies Press. 2011.

[166] C Hastie, D Mackay, et al. Vitamin D concentrations and COVID-19 infection in UK Biobank. Diab & Metab Syndrome: Clin Res Rev. 14 (4). Jul – Aug 2020. 561-565. https://www.sciencedirect.com/science/article/abs/pii/S1871402120301156?via%3Dihub

[167] H Ma, T Zhou, et al. Habitual use of vitamin D supplements and risk of coronavirus disease 2019 (COVID-19) infection a prospective study in UK Biobank. Am J Clin Nutr. Jan 29 2021. https://academic.oup.com/ajcn/advance-article/doi/10.1093/ajcn/nqaa381/6123965

[168] H Brenner. Vitamin D supplementation to prevent COVID-19 infections and deaths – accumulating evidence from epidemiological and intervention studies calls for immediate action. Nutrients. Dec 28 2020. 13 (2). 411. https://www.mdpi.com/2072-6643/13/2/411/htm#B27-nutrients-13-00411

[169] A Angelidi, M Belanger, et al. Vitamin D status is associated with in-hospital mortality and mechanical ventilation: A cohort of COVID-19 hospitalized patients. Jan 9 2021. Preprint. Mayo Clin Proc. https://www.sciencedirect.com/science/article/pii/S002561962100001X

[170] S Bennouar, A Cherif, et al. Vitamin D deficiency and low serum calcium as predictors of poor prognosis in patients with severe COVID-19. J Am Coll Nutr. Nov 22 2020. 40. 104-110. https://www.tandfonline.com/doi/full/10.1080/07315724.2020.1856013

[171] A D'Avolio, V Avataneo, et al. 25-hydroxyvitamin D concentrations are lower in patients with positive PCR for SARS-CoV-2. Nutrients. Apr 20 2020. 12 (5). https://www.mdpi.com/2072-6643/12/5/1359

[172] M Demir, F Demir, et al. Vitamin D deficiency is associated with COVID-19 positivity and severity of the disease. J Med Vir. Jan 29 2021. https://onlinelibrary.wiley.com/doi/10.1002/jmv.26832

[173] A Abdollahi, H Sarvestani, et al. The association between the level of serum 25(OH) vitamin D, obesity and underlying diseases with the risk of developing COVID-19 infection: A case-control study of hospitalized patients in Tehran, Iran. J Med Virol. Dec 12 2020. https://onlinelibrary.wiley.com/doi/10.1002/jmv.26726

[174] A Faniyi, S Lugg, et al. Vitamin D status and seroconversion for COVID-19 in UK healthcare workers. Eur. Respir J 2020. https://erj.ersjournals.com/content/erj/early/2020/11/26/13993003.04234-2020.full.pdf

[175] A Jain, R Chaurasia, et al. Analysis of vitamin D level among asymptomatic and critically ill COVID-19 patients and its correlation with inflammatory markers. Sci Rep. Nov 19 2020. 10 (1) 20191. https://pubmed.ncbi.nlm.nih.gov/33214648/

[176] A Radujkovic, T Hippchen. Vitamin D deficiency and outcome of COVID-19 patients. Nutrients. Aug 9 2020. 12 (9). 2757. https://www.mdpi.com/2072-6643/12/9/2757/htm

[177] H Susianti, C Wahono, et al. Low levels of vitamin D were associated with coagulopathy among hospitalized coronavirus (COVID-19) patients: a single-centered study in Indonesia. J Med Biochem Feb 12 2021. https://aseestant.ceon.rs/index.php/jomb/article/view/30228

[178] M Infante, A Buoso, et al. Low vitamin D status at admission as a risk factor for poor survival in hospitalized patients with COVID-19: An Italian retrospective study. J Am Coll Nutrition. Oct 31 2020. https://www.tandfonline.com/doi/full/10.1080/07315724.2021.1877580

Vitamin C vs COVID

[179] H Hemila, P Louhiala. Vitamin C may affect lung infections. Nov 1 2007. J Royal Soc Med. https://journals.sagepub.com/doi/10.1177/014107680710001109

[180] P Myint, A Wilson, et al. Plasma vitamin C concentrations and risk of incident respiratory diseases and mortality in the European Prospective Investigation into Cancer-Norfolk population-based cohort study. Jan 31 2019. Eur J Clin Nutr. https://www.nature.com/articles/s41430-019-0393-1

[181] H Hemila, P Louhiala. Vitamin C for preventing and treating pneumonia. Aug 8 2013. Cochrane DB os System Rvw. https://www.cochranelibrary.com/cdsr/doi/10.1002/14651858.CD005532.pub3/full

[182] A Glazebrook, S Thomson. The administration of vitamin C in a large institution and its effect on general health and resistance to infection. Jan 1942. Cambridge Univ Press. 42 (1). 1-19. https://www.cambridge.org/core/journals/epidemiology-and-infection/article/administration-of-vitamin-c-in-a-large-institution-and-its-effect-on-general-health-and-resistance-to-infection/E6D8D9B380FBBDB3530A81B415C70262

[183] J Kimbarowski, N Mokrow. [Colored precipitation reaction of the urine according to Kimbarowski (FARK) as an index of the effect of ascorbic acid during treatment of viral influenza. Dtsch Gesund. Dec 21 1967. 22 (51). 2413-2418. https://pubmed.ncbi.nlm.nih.gov/5614915/

[184] H Pitt, A Costrini. Vitamin C prophylaxis in marine recruits. Mar 2 1979, JAMA. 241 (9). 908-911. https://jamanetwork.com/journals/jama/article-abstract/363744

[185] F Klenner. Virus pneumonia and its treatment with vitamin C. Read by title to the Tri-State Medical Association of the Carolinas and Virginia, and in Southern Med and Surg.110(2): 36-38. Feb 1948. https://www.seanet.com/~alexs/ascorbate/194x/klenner-fr-southern_med_surg-1948-v110-n2-p36.htm

[186] Levy T (2011) Primal Panacea, Henderson, NV: MedFox Publishing. ISBN-13: 978-0983772804.

[187] Levy T (2002) Curing the Incurable. Vitamin C, Infectious Diseases, and Toxins, Henderson, NV: MedFox Publishing. ISBN-13: 978-0977952021

[188] H Hemila. Vitamin C and infections. Jan 31 2017. Nutrients. 9 (4). 339. https://www.mdpi.com/2072-6643/9/4/339

[189] Y Kim et al. Vitamin C is an essential factor on the anti-viral immune responses through the production of interferon-a/b at the initial stage of influenza A virus (H3N2) infection. Immune Netw. Apr 2020. 13(2)70-4. https://pubmed.ncbi.nlm.nih.gov/23700397/

[190] S Madhusudana, et al. In vitro inactivation of the rabies virus by ascorbic acid. Int J Infectious Dis. Jan 2004. 8(1):21-25. https://pubmed.ncbi.nlm.nih.gov/14690777/

[191] R Jariwalla et al. Antiviral and immunomodulatory activities of ascorbic acid. Subcell Biochem. 1996;25:213-31. https://pubmed.ncbi.nlm.nih.gov/8821976/

[192] A Carr et al. Vitamin C and Immune Function. Nutrients. Nov 2017; 9(11): 1211-1236. https://www.ncbi.nlm.nih.gov/pmc/articles/PMC5707683/

[193] M Gonzalez et al. High dose vitamin C and influenza: A case report. 2018. J Orthomol Medicine. 33(3). https://isom.ca/article/high-dose-vitamin-c-influenza-case-report/

[194] T Patterson, C Isales, et al. Low level of vitamin C and dysregulation of vitamin C transporter might be involved in the severity of COVID-19 infection. Aging Dis. Feb 1 2021. 12 (1). 14-26. https://pubmed.ncbi.nlm.nih.gov/33532123/

[195] A Carr, S Rowe. Factors affecting vitamin C status and prevalence of deficiency: A global health perspective. June 3 2020. Nutrients. 12 (7). https://www.mdpi.com/2072-6643/12/7/1963

[196] Y Xing, B Zhao, et al. Vitamin C supplementation is necessary for patients with coronavirus disease: An ultra-high-performance liquid chromatography-tandem mass spectrometry finding. J Pharm Biomed Anal. 196. Mar 20 2021. https://www.sciencedirect.com/science/article/pii/S073170852100039X

[197] R Schleicher, M Carroll, et al. Serum vitamin C and the prevalence of vitamin C deficiency in the United States: 2003-2004 National Health and Nutrition Examination Survey. Nov 2009. Am J Clin Nutr 90 (5). 1252-1263. https://academic.oup.com/ajcn/article/90/5/1252/4598114

[198] A Mosdol, B Erens, et al. Estimated prevalence and predictors of vitamin C deficiency within UK's low-income population. Dec 2008. J Public Health Oxf. 30 (4). 456-460. https://academic.oup.com/jpubhealth/article/30/4/456/1512595

[199] R Cheng. COVID-19, vitamin C, vaccine and integrative medicine. Apr 16 2020. Cheng Integrative Health Center Blog. https://www.drwlc.com/blog/category/covid-19-vit-c-and-integrative-medicine/

[200] Z Peng interview with R Cheng. Wuhan University. This video was removed by YouTube. However, the discussion continues on in this video, among several clinicians, in which they discuss dosing, frequency and morbidity of the patients treated. A very wide range of doses in intravenous vitamin C was used. https://youtu.be/ZfHj9FeVAJM

[201] R Cheng. Video conference with Dr ZY Peng, one of the world's first high-dose IVC trials. Apr 16 2020. Cheng Integrative Health Center Blog. https://www.drwlc.com/blog/category/covid-19-vit-c-and-integrative-medicine/

[202] J Zhang, X Rao, et al. High-dose vitamin C infusion for the treatment of critically ill COVID-19. Preprint. https://www.researchsquare.com/article/rs-52778/v2

[203] M Vizcaychipi, C Shovlin, et al. Development and implementation of a COVID-19 near real-time traffic light system in an acute hospital setting. Oct 2020. BMJ Emer Med J. 37 (10). https://emj.bmj.com/content/37/10/630

[204] ICNARC. INCARC report on COVID-19 in critical care. Jun 12 2020. https://www.patrickholford.com/uploads/2020/chelwesticnarcreportjune.pdf

[205] P Marik, P Kory et al. MATH+ protocol for the treatment of SARS-CoV-2 infection: the scientific rationale. Jul 17 2020. Exp Rev Anti-Infect Ther. 19 (2). 129-135. https://www.tandfonline.com/doi/full/10.1080/14787210.2020.1808462

[206] H Hemila, A Carr, et al. Vitamin C may increase the recovery rate of outpatient cases of SARS-CoV-2 infection by 70%: reanalysis of the COVID A to Z Randomized Clinical Trial. Preprint. https://www.researchsquare.com/article/rs-289381/v1

[207] P Kumari, S Dembra, et al. The role of vitamin C as adjuvant therapy in COVID-19. Nov 30 2020. Cureus. https://www.cureus.com/articles/45284-the-role-of-vitamin-c-as-adjuvant-therapy-in-covid-19

[208] B Zhao, Y Ling, et al Beneficial aspects of high dose intravenous vitamin C on patients with COVID-19 pneumonia in severe condition: a retrospective case series study. Ann Pall Med 10 (2). Feb 2021. https://apm.amegroups.com/article/view/56244/html

[209] A Feyaerts, W Lyten. Vitamin C as prophylaxis and adjunctive medical treatment for COVID-19? Nov-Dec 2020. Vol 79-80. Nutrition. https://www.sciencedirect.com/science/article/abs/pii/S0899900720302318?via%3Dihub

[210] D Blanco-Melo, B Nilsson-Payant, et al. Imbalanced host response to SARS-CoV-2 drives development of COVID-19. Cell. May 28 2020. 181 (5).. 1038-1045. https://www.cell.com/cell/fulltext/S0092-8674(20)30489-X?_returnURL=https%3A%2F%2Flinkinghub.elsevier.com%2Fretrieve%2Fpii%2FS009286742030489X%3Fshowall%3Dtrue

[211] R Biancatelli, M Berrill, et al. The antiviral properties of vitamin C. Sep 14 2019. Expert Rev Anti-Inf Ther. 18 (2). https://www.tandfonline.com/doi/full/10.1080/14787210.2020.1706483

[212] G Briand. COVID-19 deaths: A look at US data. Mar 18 2021. PDMJ. https://pdmj.org/papers/Briand_look_at_US_data/

[213] W Ni, X Yang. Role of angiotensin converting enzyme-2 in COVID-19. Jul 13 2020. Crit Care. 24 (422). https://www.ncbi.nlm.nih.gov/pmc/articles/PMC7356137/

[214] S Ma, S Sun, et al. Single-cell transcriptomic atlas of primate cardiopulmonary aging. Sep 10 2020. Cell Res. https://www.nature.com/articles/s41422-020-00412-6

[215] P Holford, A Carr, et al. Vitamin C- An adjunctive therapy for respiratory infection, sepsis and COVID-19. Nutrients. 12 (12). https://www.mdpi.com/2072-6643/12/12/3760/htm

[216] C Huber. Defeating cancer requires more than one treatment method: An 8-year retrospective case series using multiple nutritional and herbal agents. Keynote address to 8th Euro Global Summit on Cancer Therapy. Nov 3 2015. Valencia Spain. https://natureworksbest.com/wp-content/uploads/2019/08/Global-Cancer-Summit.pdf

[217] B Auer, D Auer, et al. The effect of ascorbic acid ingestion on the biochemical and physiochemical risk factors associated with calcium oxalate kidney stone formation. Clin Chem Lab Med. Mar 1998. 36 (3). 143-147. https://pubmed.ncbi.nlm.nih.gov/9589801/

[218] G Curhan, W Willett, et al. Intake of vitamins B6 and C and the risk of kidney stones in women. J Am Soc Nephrol. Ap[r 1999. 10 (4). 840-845. https://pubmed.ncbi.nlm.nih.gov/10203369/

[219] P Marik, P Kory et al. MATH+ protocol for the treatment of SARS-CoV-2 infection: the scientific rationale. Jul 17 2020. Exp Rev Anti-Infect Ther. 19 (2). 129-135. https://www.tandfonline.com/doi/full/10.1080/14787210.2020.1808462

Zinc versus COVID

[220] S Wuehler, J Peerson, et al. Use of national food balance data to estimate the adequacy of zinc in national food supplies: methodology and regional estimates. Jan 2 2007. Cambridge Univ Press. https://www.cambridge.org/core/journals/public-health-nutrition/article/use-of-national-food-balance-data-to-estimate-the-adequacy-of-zinc-in-national-food-supplies-methodology-and-regional-estimates/4CEBD7D6FB63A5C622FBC165A24B91D4

[221] Rink. Zinc in human health. Oct 2011. IOS Press. Vol 76 Biomedical and Health Research.

[222] A Prasad, F Beck, et al. Zinc supplementation decreases incidence of infections in the elderly: effect of zin on generation of cytokines and oxidative stress. Mar 2007. Am J Clin Nutr. 85 (3). 837-844. https://academic.oup.com/ajcn/article/85/3/837/4633003

[223] C Frederickson, J Koh, et al. Neurobiology of zinc in health and disease. July 2005. Nat Rev Neurosci. 6. 449-462. https://www.researchgate.net/publication/7849123_Frederickson_CJ_Koh_J_Y_Bush_AIThe_neurobiology_of_zinc_in_health_and_disease_Nat_Rev_Neurosci_6449-462

[224] M Lazarczyk, M Favre. Role of Zn2+ ions in host-virus interactions. Sep 9 2008. J Virol. 82 (23). 11486-11494. https://europepmc.org/article/PMC/2583646

[225] S Read, S Obeid, et al. The role of zinc in antiviral immunity. Apr 22 2019. Adv Nutr (10) 4. 696-710. https://academic.oup.com/advances/article/10/4/696/5476413

[226] T Kambe, T Tsuji, et al. The physiological, biochemical and molecular roles of zinc transporters in zinc homeostasis and metabolism. Jul 1 2015. https://journals.physiology.org/doi/full/10.1152/physrev.00035.2014

[227] I Wessels, M Maywald, et al. Zinc as a gatekeeper of immune function. Sep 27 2017. Nutrients. 9 (12). 1286. https://www.mdpi.com/2072-6643/9/12/1286/htm

[228] C Andreini, I Bertini. A bioinformatics view of zinc enzymes. Jun 2012. J Inorg Biochem. 111. 150-156. https://www.sciencedirect.com/science/article/pii/S0162013411003679?via%3Dihub

[229] J Molentin. The zinc finger-containing transcription factors GATA-4, -5 and -6: ubiquitously expressed regulators of tissue-specific gene expression. Dec 15 2000. J Biol Chem. 275 (50). 38949-38952. https://www.jbc.org/article/S0021-9258(19)55816-1/fulltext

[230] S Yamasaki, K Sakata-Sogawa, et al. Zinc is a novel intracellular second messenger. May 4 2017. J Cell Biol. 177 (4). 637-645. https://rupress.org/jcb/article/177/4/637/44755/Zinc-is-a-novel-intracellular-second-messenger

[231] D Wu, E Lewis, et al. Nutritional modulation of immune function: Analysis of evidence, mechanisms and clinical relevance. Front Immunol. Jan 15 2019. 9 (3160). https://www.ncbi.nlm.nih.gov/pmc/articles/PMC6340979/

[232] H Haase, J Ober-Blobaum, et al. Zinc signals are essential for lipopolysaccharide-induced signal transduction in monocytes. Nov 1 2008. J Immunol. 181 (9). 6491-6502. https://www.jimmunol.org/content/181/9/6491

[233] H Gao, W Dai, et al. The role of zinc and zinc homeostasis in macrophage function. J Immunol Res. Dec 6 2018. 2018 (6872621). https://www.ncbi.nlm.nih.gov/pmc/articles/PMC6304900/

[234] H Kitamura, H Morikawa, et al. Toll-like receptor-mediated regulation of zinc homeostasis influences dendritic cell function. Aug 2006. Nature Immunol. 7. 971-977. https://www.nature.com/articles/ni1373

[235] R Hasan, L Rink et al. Chelation of free ZN2+ impairs chemotaxis, phagocytosis, oxidative burst, degranulation, and cytokine production by neutrophil granulocytes. Sep 23 2015. Biol Trace Element Res 171. 790-88. https://link.springer.com/article/10.1007%2Fs12011-015-0515-0

[236] S Rajagopalan, C Winter, et al. The Ig-related killer cell inhibitory receptor binds zinc and requires zinc for recognition of HLA-C on target cells. Nov 1 1995. J Immunol. 155 (9). 4143-4146. https://pubmed.ncbi.nlm.nih.gov/7594568/

[237] S Kumar, S Rajagopalan, et al. Zinc-induced polymerization of killer cell Ig-like receptor into filaments promotes it inhibitory function at cytotoxic immunological synapses. Apr 7 2016. Mol Cell 62 (1). P21-33. https://www.cell.com/molecular-cell/fulltext/S1097-2765(16)00187-8?_returnURL=https%3A%2F%2Flinkinghub.elsevier.com%2Fretrieve%2Fpii%2FS1097276516001878%3Fshowall%3Dtrue

[238] P Fraker. Roles for cell death in zinc deficiency. Mar 2005. J Nutr. 135 (3). 359-362. https://pubmed.ncbi.nlm.nih.gov/15735063/

[239] I Wessels, M Maywald, et al. Zinc as a gatekeeper of immune function. Sep 27 2017. Nutrients. 9 (12). 1286. https://www.mdpi.com/2072-6643/9/12/1286/htm

[240] M Dardenne, W Savino, et al. In vivo and in vitro studies of thymulin in marginally zinc-deficient mice. Eur J Immunol. 14 (5). 454-458. https://onlinelibrary.wiley.com/doi/abs/10.1002/eji.1830140513

[241] P Fraker, L King. Reprogramming of the immune system during zinc deficiency. Feb 6 2004. Ann Rev Nutr. 24. 277-298. https://www.annualreviews.org/doi/10.1146/annurev.nutr.24.012003.132454

[242] T Miyai, S Hojyo, et al. Zinc transporter SLC39A10/ZIP10 facilitates antiapoptotic signaling during early B-cell development. Aug 12 2014. Proc Natl Acad Sci. 111 (32). 11780-11785. https://www.pnas.org/content/111/32/11780

[243] I Wessels, M Maywald, et al. Zinc as a gatekeeper of immune function. Sep 27 2017. Nutrients. 9 (12). 1286. https://www.mdpi.com/2072-6643/9/12/1286/htm

[244] S Read, S Obeid, et al. The role of zinc in antiviral immunity. Apr 22 2019. Adv Nutr. 10 (4). 696-710. https://academic.oup.com/advances/article/10/4/696/5476413

[245] A te Velthuis, S van den Worm, et al. Zn(2+) inhibits coronavirus and arterivirus RNA polymerase activity in vitro and zinc ionophores block the replication of these viruses in cell culture. Nov 4 2010. PLoS Path 6 (11). https://journals.plos.org/plospathogens/article?id=10.1371/journal.ppat.1001176

[246] A te Velthuis, S van den Worm, et al. Zn(2+) inhibits coronavirus and arterivirus RNA polymerase activity in vitro and zinc ionophores block the replication of these viruses in cell culture. Nov 4 2010. PLoS Path 6 (11). https://journals.plos.org/plospathogens/article?id=10.1371/journal.ppat.1001176

[247] M Cordingley, R Register, et al. Cleavage of small peptides in vitro by human rhinovirus 14 3C protease expressed in Escherichia coli. J Viro. Nov 30 1989. 63 (12). 5037-5045. https://europepmc.org/article/PMC/251164

[248] M Denison, S Perlman. Translation and processing of mouse hepatitis virus virion RNA in a cell-free system. Sep 30 1986. J Virol. 60 (1). 12-18. https://europepmc.org/article/PMC/253896

[249] M Denison, P Zoltick et al. Intracellular processing of the N-terminal ORF 1a proteins of the coronavirus MHV-A59 requires multiple proteolytic events. Jul 1992. Virology. 189 (1). 274-284. https://europepmc.org/article/MED/1318604

[250] A te Velthuis, S van den Worm, et al. Zn(2+) inhibits coronavirus and arterivirus RNA polymerase activity in vitro and zinc ionophores block the replication of these viruses in cell culture. Nov 4 2010. PLoS Path 6 (11). https://journals.plos.org/plospathogens/article?id=10.1371/journal.ppat.1001176

[251] World Health Organization. The World Health Report 2002. 2003. Midwifery. 19. 72-73. doi: 10.1054/midw.2002.0343

[252] I Wessels, B Rolles, et al. The potential impact of zinc supplementation on COVID-19 pathogenesis. Front Immunol. Jul 10 2020. https://www.frontiersin.org/articles/10.3389/fimmu.2020.01712/full#B10

[253] J Hamming, W Timens, et al. Tissue distribution of ACE2 protein, the functional receptor for SARS coronavirus. A first step in understanding SARS pathogenesis. Jan 30 2004. J Path. 203. 631-637. https://onlinelibrary.wiley.com/doi/pdf/10.1002/path.1570

[254] E Roscioli, H Jersmann, et al. Zinc deficiency as a codeterminant for airway epithelial barrier dysfunction in an ex vivo model of COPD. Aug 20 2017. Int J COPD. 2017 (12). 3503-3510. https://www.dovepress.com/zinc-deficiency-as-a-codeterminant--for-airway-epithelial-barrier-dysf-peer-reviewed-article-COPD

[255] A Darma, A Athiyyah, et al. Zinc supplementation effect on the bronchial cilia length, the number of cilia, and the number of intact bronchial cells in zinc deficiency rats. 2020. Indo Biomed J. 12 (1). https://inabj.org/index.php/ibj/article/view/998

[256] I Wessels, B Rolles, et al. The potential impact of zinc supplementation on COVID-19 pathogenesis. Front Immunol. Jul 10 2020. https://www.frontiersin.org/articles/10.3389/fimmu.2020.01712/full#B10

[257] A Prasad. Effects of zinc deficiency on Th1 and Th2 cytokine shifts. Sep 1 2000. J Infect Dis. 182 (1). https://academic.oup.com/jid/article/182/Supplement_1/S62/2191506

[258] P Zalewski, A Truong-Tran, et al. Zinc metabolism in airway epithelium and airway inflammation: basic mechanisms and clinical targets: A review. Feb 2005. Pharmacol. Ther. 105 (2). 127-149. https://pubmed.ncbi.nlm.nih.gov/15670623/

[259] N Cvijanovich, J King, et al. Zinc homeostasis in pediatric critical illness. Pediatr Crit Care Med. Jan 2009. 10 (1). 29-34. https://pubmed.ncbi.nlm.nih.gov/19057435/

[260] H Wong, T Shanley, et al. Genome-level expression in pediatric septic shock indicate a role for altered zinc homeostasis in poor outcome. Aug 2007. Physiolog Genomics. 30 (2). 146-155. https://www.researchgate.net/publication/6432274_Genome-level_expression_profiles_in_pediatric_septic_shock_indicate_a_role_for_altered_zinc_homeostasis_in_poor_outcome

[261] R Heller, Q Sun, et al. Prediction of survival odds in COVID-19 by zinc, age and selenoprotein P as composite biomarker. Jan 2021. Redox Biol. 38. 101764. https://www.sciencedirect.com/science/article/pii/S2213231720309691#bib79

[262] Y Yasui, H Yasui, et al. Analysis of the predictive factors for a critical illness of COVID-19 during treatment – relationship between serum zinc level and critical illness of COVID-19. Sep 7 2020. Intl J Inf Dis. 100. 230-236. https://www.ijidonline.com/article/S1201-9712(20)30723-2/fulltext

[263] D Jothimani, E Kailasam, et al. COVID-19: Poor outcomes in patients with zinc deficiency. Sep 10 2020. Intl J Inf Dis. 100. 343-349. https://www.ijidonline.com/article/S1201-9712(20)30730-X/fulltext

[264] G Dubourg, J Lagier, et al. Low blood zinc concentrations in patients with poor clinical outcome during SARS-CoV-2 infection: is there a need to supplement with zinc COVID-19 patients? Feb 13 2021. J Microbiol Immunol Infect. S1684-1182 (21). 26-28. https://pubmed.ncbi.nlm.nih.gov/33632620/

[265] A Stoll. Zinc salts for the treatment of olfactory and gustatory symptoms in psychiatric patients: a case series. J Clin Psychaitry. Jul 1994. 55(7): 309-11. https://pubmed.ncbi.nlm.nih.gov/7915275/

[266] K Jiang. How COVID-19 causes loss of sense of smell. Harvard University. Jul 24 2020. https://hms.harvard.edu/news/how-covid-19-causes-loss-smell

[267] Eurosurveillance ET. Updated rapid risk assessment from ECDC on coronavirus disease 2019 (COVID-19) pandemic: increased transmission in the EU/EEA and the UK. March 12 2020. Euro Surveill. https://www.eurosurveillance.org/content/10.2807/1560-7917.ES.2020.25.10.2003121

[268] M Rukgauer, J Klein, et al. Reference values for the trace elements copper, manganese, selenium and zinc in the serum / plasma of children, adolescents and adults. 1997. J Trace Elements Med Biol. 11 (2). 92-98. https://www.sciencedirect.com/science/article/abs/pii/S0946672X97800326?via%3Dihub

[269] G Kumel, S Schrader, et al. The mechanism of the antiherpetic activity of zinc sulphate. Dec 1 1990. J Gen Vir. 71 (12). https://www.microbiologyresearch.org/content/journal/jgv/10.1099/0022-1317-71-12-2989

Zinc and Hydroxychloroquine versus COVID

[270] US Centers for Disease Control and Prevention (CDC) https://www.cdc.gov/parasites/malaria/index.html

[271] S Gold. White paper on hydroxychloroquine. White paper on HCQ 2020.2.pdf https://drive.google.com/file/d/1-gsn_Ye2EYDDkV_79Ag1tgUqZLNCMSt-/view

[272] B Yeo. [peer-reviewed study] in A Manual of Medical Treatment or Clinical Therapeutics. 1901. https://archive.org/details/b21303629_0002/page/656/mode/2up?ref=ol&view=theater

[273] M Vincent, E Bergeron, et al. Chloroquine is a potent inhibitor of SARS coronavirus infection and spread. Aug 22 2005. Virol J 2 (69). https://www.ncbi.nlm.nih.gov/pmc/articles/PMC1232869/

[274] H Bailey. Edwin Wiley Grove 1850-1927. Tennessee Encyclopedia. https://tennesseeencyclopedia.net/entries/edwin-wiley-grove/

[275] A Savarino, L Di Trani, et al. New insights into the antiviral effects of chloroquine. Feb 1 2006. The Lancet. 6 (2). 67-69. https://www.thelancet.com/journals/laninf/article/PIIS1473-3099(06)70361-9/fulltext

[276] M Al-Bari. Targeting endosomal acidification by chloroquine analogs as a promising strategy for the treatment of emerging viral diseases. Jan 22 2017. Pharm Res Perspec. 5 (1). E00293. https://europepmc.org/article/PMC/5461643

[277] J Rolain, P Colson, et al. Recycling of chloroquine and its hydroxyl analogue to face bacterial, fungal and viral infections in the 21st century. Int J Antimicrob Agents. 30 (4). Oct 2007. 297-308. https://www.sciencedirect.com/science/article/abs/pii/S0924857907002580

[278] A Kaufmann, J Krise. Lysosomal sequestration of amine-containing drugs: analysis and therapeutic implications. Apr 1 2007. J Pharm Sci. 96 (4). 729-746. https://jpharmsci.org/article/S0022-3549(16)32230-4/fulltext

[279] M Degtyarev, A De Mazière, et al. Akt inhibition promotes autophagy and sensitizes PTEN-null tumors to lysosomotropic agents. Sep 30 2008. J Cell Biol 183 (1). 101-116. https://europepmc.org/article/PMC/2557046

[280] N Yang, H Shen. Targeting the endocytic pathway and autophagy process as a novel therapeutic strategy in COVID-19. 2020. Int J Biol Sci. 16 (10). 1724-1731. https://www.ijbs.com/v16p1724.htm#B45

[281] P D'Adamo. COVID-19: chloroquine, zinc and quercitin. People, Nature and Data Apr 7 2020. https://dadamo.com/dangerous/2020/04/07/covid-19-chloroquine-zinc-and-quercetin/

[282] R Derwand, M Scholz. Does zinc supplementation enhance the clinical efficacy of chloroquine / hydroxychloroquine to win today's battle against COVID-19? Sep 2020. Med Hypotheses. 142 (109815). https://www.sciencedirect.com/science/article/pii/S0306987720306435#b0055

[283] J Kearney. Chloroquine as a potential treatment and prevention measure for the 2019 novel coronavirus: a review. March 16 2020. Preprints. 202003027. https://www.preprints.org/manuscript/202003.0275/v1

[284] Z Yang, Y Huang, et al. pH-dependent entry of severe acute respiratory syndrome coronavirus is mediated by the spike glycoprotein and enhanced by dendritic cell transfer through DC-SIGN. Dec 2003. J Virology https://jvi.asm.org/content/78/11/5642/article-info

[285] G Simmons, J Reeves, et al. Characterization of severe acute respiratory syndrome-associated coronavirus (SARS-CoV) spike glycoprotein-mediated viral entry. Mar 9 2004. Proc Natl Acad Sci. 101 (12). 4240-4245. https://www.ncbi.nlm.nih.gov/pmc/articles/PMC384725/

[286] N Yang, H Shen. Targeting the endocytic pathway and autophagy process as a novel therapeutic strategy in COVID-19. 2020. Int J Biol Sci. 16 (10). 1724-1731. https://www.ijbs.com/v16p1724.htm#B45

[287] J Xue, A Moyer, et al. Chloroquine is a zinc ionophore. Oct 1 2014. PLoS One. https://journals.plos.org/plosone/article?id=10.1371/journal.pone.0109180

[288] J Xue, A Moyer, et al. Chloroquine is a zinc ionophore. Oct 1 2014. PLoS One. https://journals.plos.org/plosone/article?id=10.1371/journal.pone.0109180

[289] M Dang, J Song. Structural basis of anti-SARS-CoV-2 activity of hydroxychloroquine: specific binding to NTD/CTD and disruption of LLPS on N protein. Mar 17 2021. BioRxIV. https://www.biorxiv.org/content/10.1101/2021.03.16.435741v1.full

[290] R Derwand, M Scholz. Does zinc supplementation enhance the clinical efficacy of chloroquine / hydroxychloroquine to win today's battle against COVID-19? Sep 2020. Med Hypotheses. 142. 109815. https://www.sciencedirect.com/science/article/pii/S0306987720306435#b0105

[291] V Zelenko. Nebulized hydroxychloroquine for COVID-19 treatment: 80x improvement in breathing. Jan 24 2021. Preprint. https://docs.google.com/document/d/1WjfphkNfYDxF4MMw7bS9HJpmeGuhwEFuJkUTexjHHOc/edit

[292] J Lagier, M Million, et al. Outcomes of 3,737 COVID-19 patients treated with hydroxychloroquine/azithromycin and other regiments in Marseille, France: A retrospective analysis. Jul Aug 2020. Travel Med Inf Dis. 36 (101791). https://www.sciencedirect.com/science/article/pii/S1477893920302817

[293] H Risch. Opinion: Early outpatient treatment of symptomatic high-risk COVID-19 patients that should be ramped-up immediately as key to the pandemic crisis. Amer J Epidem May 27 2020. https://academic.oup.com/aje/advance-article/doi/10.1093/aje/kwaa093/5847586

[294] S Bhandari. HCQ beneficial as preventive drug: SMS doctors told ICMR. Jun 19 2020. SMS Medical College. Reported in Healthworld. https://health.economictimes.indiatimes.com/news/diagnostics/hcq-beneficial-as-preventive-drug-sms-doctors-told-icmr/76464620

[295] S Bhandari, G Rankawat, et al. A preventive study on hydroxychloroquine prophylaxis against COVID-19 in health care workers at a tertiary care center in North India. Jul 19 2020. Int J Med Pub Health. 11 (1): 24-27. https://ijmedph.org/sites/default/files/IntJMedPubHealth-11-1-24.pdf

[296] N Dev, R Meena, et al. Risk factors and frequency of COVID-19 among healthcare workers at a tertiary care centre in India: a case-control study. Mar 24 2021. Transactions Royal Soc Trop Med Hyg. https://academic.oup.com/trstmh/advance-article/doi/10.1093/trstmh/trab047/6186057

[297] R Derwand, M Scholz, et al. COVID-19 outpatients: early risk-stratified treatment with zinc plus low-dose hydroxychloroquine and azithromycin: a retrospecitive case series study. Dec 2020. 56 (6). 106214. https://www.sciencedirect.com/science/article/pii/S0924857920304258

[298] M Scholz et al. COVID-19 outpatients - Early risk-stratified treatment with zinc plus low dose hydroxychloroquine and azithromycin: A retrospective case series study. Jun 30 2020. https://www.preprints.org/manuscript/202007.0025/v1

[299] J Frontera, J Rahimian, et al. Treatment with zinc is associated with reduced in-hospital mortality among COVID-19 patients: A multi-center cohort study. Oct 26 2020. BMC Infectious Diseases. https://www.researchsquare.com/article/rs-94509/v1

[300] S Hatfill. An effective COVID treatment the media continues to besmirch: Analysis. Real Clear Politics. Aug 4 2020. https://www.realclearpolitics.com/articles/2020/08/04/an_effective_covid_treatment_the_media_continues_to_besmirch_143875.html

[301] Graph accompanies Dr.Hatfill'sarticle. Ibid. http://assets.realclear.com/images/51/517550_5_.png

[302] H Risch interview with Mark Levin. Fox News. Aug 24 2020. https://www.bitchute.com/video/mAOVVqNfbXyT/

[303] Covid Analysis. HCQ is effective for COVID-19 when used early: Real time meta-analysis of 219 studies. Oct 20 2020. Updated Mar 13 2021. HCQ Meta. https://hcqmeta.com/

[304] https://c19study.com

[305] H Dabbagh-Bazarbachi, et al. Zinc ionophore activity of quercitin and epigallocatechin-gallate (EGCG): from Hepa 1-6 cells to a liposome model. J Agric Food Chem. Jul 22 2014.62(32): 8085-8093. https://pubs.acs.org/doi/10.1021/jf5014633

[306] W Wu. Quercitin as an antiviral agent inhibits influenza A virus (IAV) entry. Viruses. Jan2016. 8(1). https://www.ncbi.nlm.nih.gov/pmc/articles/PMC4728566/

[307] Op cit. H Dabbagh-Bazarbachi, et al. https://pubs.acs.org/doi/10.1021/jf5014633

[308] K Kaihatsu, et al. Antiviral mechanism of action of epigallocatechin-3-O-gallate and its fatty acid esters. Molecules. 2018. 23(10):2475. https://doi.org/10.3390/molecules23102475. https://www.mdpi.com/1420-3049/23/10/2475/htm

Ivermectin vs COVID

[309] K Sharun, K Dhama, et al. Ivermectin, a new candidate therapeutic against SARS-CoV-2/COVID-19. May 30 2020. Ann Clin Microbiol Antimicrob. 19 (23). https://ann-clinmicrob.biomedcentral.com/articles/10.1186/s12941-020-00368-w

[310] Covid Analysis. Ivermectin is effective for COVID-19: Real-time meta-analysis of 49 studies. Nov 26 2020. Updated Mar 31 2021. https://ivmmeta.com/

[311] J Rajter, M Sherman, et al. Use of ivermectin is associated with lower mortality in hospitalized patients with coronavirus disease 2019: The ivermectin in COVID nineteen study. Jan 2021. Chest. 159 (1). 85-92. https://www.sciencedirect.com/science/article/pii/S0012369220348984

[312] R Chahla, L Ruiz, et al. Ivermectin repurposing for COVID-19 treatment of outpatients in mild stage in primary health care centers. Mar 30 2021. MedRxiv. https://www.medrxiv.org/content/10.1101/2021.03.29.21254554v1

[313] H Tanioka, S Tanioka, et al. Why COVID-19 is not so spread in Africa: How does Ivermectin affect it? Mar 26 2021. MedRXiv. https://www.medrxiv.org/content/10.1101/2021.03.26.21254377v1.full-text

[314] T Jabeen, M Khader, et al. A review on the antiparasitic drug ivermectin for various viral infections and possibilities of using it for novel severe acute respiratory syndrome coronavirus 2: New hope to treat coronavirus disease – 2019. Jun 2020. Asian J Pharm Clin Res. https://www.researchgate.net/publication/343742900_A_REVIEW_ON_THE_ANTIPARASITIC_DRUG_IVERMECTIN_FOR_VARIOUS_VIRAL_INFECTIONS_AND_POSSIBILITIES_OF_USING_IT_FOR_NOVEL_SEVERE_ACUTE_RESPIRATORY_SYNDROME_CORONAVIRUS_2_NEW_HOPE_TO_TREAT_CORONAVIRUS_DISEASE

[315] J Sanz-Navarro, C Feal, et al. Treatment of human scabies with oral ivermectin. Sep 2017. Actas Dermos. 108 (7). 643-649. https://pubmed.ncbi.nlm.nih.gov/28385424/

[316] J Remme, R Baker, et al. A community trial of ivermectin in the onchocerciasis focus of Asubende, Ghana. I: Effect on the microfilarial reservoir and the transmission of Onchocerca volvulus. Sep 1989. Trop Med Parasitol. 40 (3). 367-374. https://pubmed.ncbi.nlm.nih.gov/2617046/

[317] M Pacqué, B Muñoz, et al. Pregnancy outcome after inadvertent ivermectin treatment during community-based distribution. Dec 15 1990. Lancet. 336 (8729). 1486-1489. https://pubmed.ncbi.nlm.nih.gov/1979100/

[318] US FDA. FAQ: COVID-19 and ivermectin intended for animals. Dec 16 2020. https://www.fda.gov/animal-veterinary/product-safety-information/faq-covid-19-and-ivermectin-intended-animals

[319] R Croci, E Bottaro, et al. Liposomal systems as nanocarriers for the antiviral agent ivermectin. May 8 2016. Int J Biomater. https://www.ncbi.nlm.nih.gov/pmc/articles/PMC4875998/

[320] M Yagisawa, P Foster, et al. Global trends in clinical studies of ivermectin in COVID-19. Mar 10 2021. Japanese J Antibiotics. 74 (1). 44-95. http://jja-contents.wdc-jp.com/pdf/JJA74/74-1-open/74-1_44-95.pdf

[321] L Caly, J Druce, et al. The FDA-approved drug ivermectin inhibits the replication of SARS-CoV-2 in vitro. Jun 2020. Antiviral Res. https://www.sciencedirect.com/science/article/pii/S0166354220302011?via%3Dihub

[322] M Turkia. A timeline of ivermectin-related events in the COVID-19 pandemic. Mar 2021. https://www.researchgate.net/publication/350496335_A_Timeline_of_Ivermectin-Related_Events_in_the_COVID-19_Pandemic

[323] I Udofia, K Gbayo, et al. In silico studies of selected multi-drug targeting against 3CLpro and nsp12 RNA-dependent RNA-polymerase proteins of SARS-CoV-2 and SARS-CoV. Mar 25 2021. Network Mod Anal Health Inf Bioinf. 10 (22). https://link.springer.com/article/10.1007/s13721-021-00299-2

[324] L Caly, J Druce, et al. The FDA-approved drug ivermectin inhibits the replication of SARS-CoV-2 in vitro. Jun 2020. Antiviral Res. https://www.sciencedirect.com/science/article/pii/S0166354220302011?via%3Dihub

[325] M Tay, J Fraser, et al. Nuclear localization of dengue (DENV) 1-4 non-structural protein 5; protection against all 4 DENV serotypes by the inhibitor ivermectin. Sep 2013. Antivir Res. 99 (3). 301-306. https://www.sciencedirect.com/science/article/abs/pii/S0166354213001599

[326] K Wagstaff, H Sivakumaran, et al. Ivermectin is a specific inhibitor of importin alpha/beta-mediated nuclear import able to inhibit replication of HIV-1 and dengue virus. May 1 2012. J Biochem. 443 (3). 851-856. https://www.ncbi.nlm.nih.gov/pmc/articles/PMC3327999/

[327] S Yang, S Atkinson, et al. The broad spectrum antiviral ivermectin targets the host nuclear transport importin alpha/beta1 heterodimer. May 2020. Antivir Res. 104760. https://www.sciencedirect.com/science/article/abs/pii/S0166354219307211

[328] A Choudhury, N Das, et al. Exploring the binding efficacy of ivermectin against the key proteins of SARS-CoV-2 pathogenesis: an in silico approach. Future Vir. Mar 25 2021. https://www.futuremedicine.com/doi/10.2217/fvl-2020-0342

[329] M Yagisawa, P Foster, et al. Global trends in clinical studies of ivermectin in COVID-19. Mar 10 2021. Japanese J Antibiotics. 74 (1). 44-95. http://jja-contents.wdc-jp.com/pdf/JJA74/74-1-open/74-1_44-95.pdf

Lockdowns

[330] J Bote. At least 22 states pause reopening or take new steps to limit the spread of COVID-19. USA Today. Jun 30 2020. https://www.usatoday.com/storytelling/coronavirus-reopening-america-map/

[331] US Centers for Disease Control and Prevention. Daily updates of totals by week and state. Provisional death counts for coronavirus disease 2019 (COVID-19). National Center for Health Statistics. https://www.cdc.gov/nchs/nvss/vsrr/COVID19/

Provisional Death Counts for Co ×

cdc.gov/nchs/nvss/vsrr/COVID19/

Google New Tab

Table 1. Deaths involving coronavirus disease 2019 (COVID-19), pneumonia, and influenz reported to NCHS by week ending date, United States. Week ending 2/1/2020 to 6/6/2020.*

Updated June 12, 2020

Week ending date in which the death occurred	All Deaths involving COVID-19 (U07.1)[1]	Deaths from All Causes	Percent of Expected Deaths[2]	Deaths involving Pneumonia, with or without COVID-19, excluding Influenza deaths (J12.0–J18.9)[3]	Deaths involving COVID-19 and Pneumonia, excluding Influenza (U07.1 and J12.0–J18.9)[3]	All Deaths involving Influenza, with or without COVID-19 or Pneumonia (J09–J11), includes COVID-19 or Pneumonia[4]
Total Deaths	**98,695**	1,116,797	104	109,291	42,863	6,401
2/1/2020	1	57,815	97	3,738	0	476
2/8/2020	1	58,356	98	3,725	0	514
2/15/2020	0	57,698	98	3,755	0	544
2/22/2020	4	57,800	100	3,631	1	557
2/29/2020	5	58,177	101	3,755	3	636
3/7/2020	32	58,433	101	3,884	16	619
3/14/2020	52	57,307	100	3,874	27	608
3/21/2020	547	57,919	102	4,450	245	539
3/28/2020	3,036	61,841	111	6,020	1,370	438
4/4/2020	9,462	70,290	126	9,571	4,529	460
4/11/2020	15,610	76,652	138	11,632	6,998	464
4/18/2020	16,207	73,807	136	10,872	6,935	258
4/25/2020	13,922	69,565	129	9,549	5,968	142
5/2/2020	11,389	64,159	119	8,039	4,838	57
5/9/2020	10,262	61,368	116	7,198	4,357	45
5/16/2020	8,089	57,287	109	6,024	3,378	18
5/23/2020	5,673	51,381	98	4,814	2,430	15

[332] J Burn-Murdoch, V Romei, et al. Global coronavirus death toll could be 60% higher than reported. Financial Times. Apr 26 2020. https://www.ft.com/content/6bd88b7d-3386-4543-b2e9-0d5c6fac846c

[333] T Meunier. Full lockdown policies in western Europe countries have no evident impacts on the COVID-19 epidemic. MedRxIV. Preprint May 1 2020. https://doi.org/10.1101/2020.04.24.20078717. https://www.medrxiv.org/content/10.1101/2020.04.24.20078717v1

[334] T Rodgers. Do lockdowns save many lives? In most places the data says no. Wall Street Journal. Apr 26 2020. https://www.wsj.com/articles/do-lockdowns-save-many-lives-is-most-places-the-data-say-no-11587930911

[335] G Zhuang, M Shen, et al. Potential false-positive rate among the 'asymptomatic infected individuals' in close contacts of COVID-19 patients. ResearchGate. Mar 2020. https://www.researchgate.net/publication/339770271_Potential_false-positive_rate_among_the_%27asymptomatic_infected_individuals%27_in_close_contacts_of_COVID-19_patients

[336] D Crowe. Op-Ed: Does the 2019 coronavirus exist? GreenMed Info. Mar 14 2020. https://www.greenmedinfo.com/blog/does-2019-coronavirus-exist

[337] US Centers for Disease Control and Prevention. ICD-10-CM official coding and reporting guidelines, April 1, 2020 through September 30, 2020. https://www.cdc.gov/nchs/data/icd/COVID-19-guidelines-final.pdf

[338] Accounting Weekly. US hospitals getting paid to list patients as Covid-19. Apr 11 2020. https://accountingweekly.com/us-hospitals-getting-paid-to-list-patients-as-covid-19/

[339] US Centers for Disease Control and Prevention. Daily updates of totals by week and state. Provisional death counts for coronavirus disease 2019 (COVID-19). National Center for Health Statistics. https://www.cdc.gov/nchs/nvss/vsrr/COVID19/

[340] CDC data is as follows, with screenprints from https://www.cdc.gov/nchs/nvss/vsrr/COVID19/ for each of the respective dates below.

CDC data for May 15, 2020, part 1 of 4

cdc.gov/nchs/nvss/vsrr/COVID19/

Table 2. Deaths involving coronavirus disease 2019 (COVID-19), pneumonia, and influenza reported to NCHS by jurisdiction of occurrence, United States. Week ending 2/1/2020 to 5/9/2020.*

Updated May 15, 2020

Jurisdiction of Occurrence	COVID-19 Deaths (U07.1)[1]	Deaths from All Causes	Percent of Expected Deaths[2]	Pneumonia Deaths (J12.0–J18.9)[3]	Deaths with Pneumonia and COVID-19 (J12.0–J18.9 and U07.1)[3]	Influenza Deaths (J09–J11)[4]	Deaths with Pneumonia, Influenza, or COVID-19 U07.1 or J09–J18.9)[5]
United States[6]	**60,299**	857,948	101	81,318	26,516	6,158	120,370
Alabama	**342**	14,849	95	955	94	87	1,289
Alaska	-	1,034	83	49	-	-	58
Arizona	**401**	18,648	103	1,350	191	108	1,668
Arkansas	**57**	9,075	96	629	17	71	740
California	**1,904**	80,587	99	7,113	1,113	557	8,461
Colorado	**878**	12,853	109	1,219	486	92	1,698
Connecticut	**525**	3,503	37	315	118	47	768
Delaware	**162**	2,549	93	193	62	15	308
District of Columbia	**161**	1,823	101	286	161	-	293
Florida	**1,477**	63,846	102	4,824	777	295	5,814
Georgia	**935**	23,893	95	1,744	432	100	2,347
Hawaii	**15**	3,318	96	221	-	19	250

CDC data for May 15, 2020, part 2 of 4

cdc.gov/nchs/nvss/vsrr/COVID19/

Georgia	**935**	23,893	95	1,744	432	100	2,347
Hawaii	**15**	3,318	96	221	-	19	250
Idaho	**66**	4,170	99	224	21	24	293
Illinois	**2,245**	34,358	109	3,466	1,200	173	4,681
Indiana	**1,088**	20,130	102	1,983	509	125	2,685
Iowa	**188**	8,666	96	618	39	82	849
Kansas	**132**	7,715	97	540	59	86	699
Kentucky	**207**	12,684	88	1,155	109	91	1,344
Louisiana	**1,497**	13,862	103	1,272	670	68	2,162
Maine	**61**	4,397	101	353	15	31	430
Maryland	**1,320**	16,383	110	1,594	493	118	2,524
Massachusetts	**4,108**	22,373	125	3,033	1,492	155	5,797
Michigan	**3,361**	32,764	113	3,674	1,682	231	5,580
Minnesota	**469**	13,466	103	1,009	136	116	1,457
Mississippi	**334**	9,518	102	886	152	51	1,119
Missouri	**380**	17,936	93	1,167	130	170	1,587
Montana	15	2,707	88	157	-	33	203
Nebraska	**42**	4,520	89	350	10	27	409
Nevada	**237**	7,573	98	684	182	38	777
New Hampshire	**117**	3,753	102	271	32	30	385

CDC data for May 15, 2020, part 3 of 4

Death Counts for Co × G influenza deaths per year US - G × | +

cdc.gov/nchs/nvss/vsrr/COVID19/

New Hampshire	**117**	3,753	102	271	32	30	385
New Jersey	**7,237**	31,292	141	5,545	3,592	112	9,292
New Mexico	**148**	5,161	93	388	68	27	495
New York[7]	**7,267**	38,394	129	6,528	3,675	199	10,303
New York City	**15,440**	37,759	236	8,079	5,871	928	17,779
North Carolina	**145**	15,431	54	971	57	177	1,236
North Dakota	**17**	1,743	83	160	-	19	190
Ohio	**797**	33,082	90	2,104	348	241	2,794
Oklahoma	**193**	10,149	85	930	76	99	1,143
Oregon	**119**	10,093	93	541	47	61	674
Pennsylvania	**2,819**	35,445	87	2,984	1,065	182	4,917
Rhode Island	**205**	2,784	88	215	72	24	372
South Carolina	**220**	14,778	102	911	79	94	1,146
South Dakota	**21**	2,203	90	172	-	21	205
Tennessee	**204**	21,581	98	1,612	93	122	1,845
Texas	**745**	57,248	96	4,295	319	321	5,040
Utah	**57**	5,628	101	321	21	40	397
Vermont	**47**	1,753	102	116	11	14	166
Virginia	**744**	21,243	104	1,292	259	109	1,884
Washington	**747**	16,242	95	1,403	398	102	1,850

CDC data for May 15, 2020, part 4 of 4

cdc.gov/nchs/nvss/vsrr/COVID19/

Ohio	[illegible]	[illegible]	[illegible]	[illegible]	[illegible]	[illegible]	[illegible]
Oklahoma	193	10,149	85	930	76	99	1,143
Oregon	119	10,093	93	541	47	61	674
Pennsylvania	2,819	35,445	87	2,984	1,065	182	4,917
Rhode Island	205	2,784	88	215	72	24	372
South Carolina	220	14,778	102	911	79	94	1,146
South Dakota	21	2,203	90	172	-	21	205
Tennessee	204	21,581	98	1,612	93	122	1,845
Texas	745	57,248	96	4,295	319	321	5,040
Utah	57	5,628	101	321	21	40	397
Vermont	47	1,753	102	116	11	14	166
Virginia	744	21,243	104	1,292	259	109	1,884
Washington	747	16,242	95	1,403	398	102	1,850
West Virginia	36	5,513	81	407	-	57	493
Wisconsin	355	16,160	103	908	47	147	1,361
Wyoming	-	1,313	98	102	-	-	113
Puerto Rico	98	6,298	74	897	50	36	981

NOTE: Number of deaths reported in this table are the total number of deaths received and coded as of the date of analysis and do not represent all deaths that occurred in that period.

*Data during this period are incomplete because of the lag in time between when the death occurred and when the death certificate is completed, submitted to NCHS and processed for reporting purposes. This delay can range from 1 week to 8 weeks or more, depending on the jurisdiction, age, and cause of death.

[1]Deaths with confirmed or presumed COVID-19, coded to ICD-10 code U07.1.

[2]Percent of expected deaths is the number of deaths for all causes for this week in 2020 compared to the average number across the

CDC data for May 22, 2020, part 1 of 3

Provisional Death Counts for Co × +

cdc.gov/nchs/nvss/vsrr/COVID19/

Google

Table 2. Deaths involving coronavirus disease 2019 (COVID-19), pneumonia, and influer NCHS by jurisdiction of occurrence, United States. Week ending 2/1/2020 to 5/16/2020.*

Updated May 22, 2020

Jurisdiction of Occurrence	COVID-19 Deaths (U07.1)[1]	Deaths from All Causes	Percent of Expected Deaths[2]	Pneumonia Deaths (J12.0–J18.9)[3]	Deaths with Pneumonia and COVID-19 (J12.0–J18.9 and U07.1)[3]	Influenza Deaths (J09–J11)[4]
United States[6]	**73,639**	922,510	103	89,555	32,320	6,253
Alabama	**423**	15,836	95	1,023	120	88
Alaska	-	1,125	85	54	-	-
Arizona	**518**	19,997	105	1,483	254	109
Arkansas	**82**	9,842	98	673	22	74
California	**2,485**	86,030	100	7,718	1,414	562
Colorado	**1,088**	13,815	111	1,361	588	93
Connecticut	**918**	4,875	48	438	195	56
Delaware	**217**	2,758	96	220	85	15
District of Columbia	**216**	1,962	103	344	216	-
Florida	**1,698**	67,473	102	5,135	889	300
Georgia	**1,139**	25,493	97	1,895	530	102
Hawaii	**15**	3,538	97	236	-	19
Idaho	**70**	4,362	98	227	23	24

CDC data for May 22, 2020, part 2 of 3

Provisional Death Counts for Co

cdc.gov/nchs/nvss/vsrr/COVID19/

Google

Idaho	70	4,362	98	227	23	24
Illinois	3,016	37,267	112	3,986	1,601	174
Indiana	1,396	21,367	102	2,149	629	126
Iowa	264	9,244	97	662	62	83
Kansas	163	8,126	97	574	73	87
Kentucky	274	13,570	90	1,243	141	93
Louisiana	1,754	14,889	105	1,411	778	70
Maine	70	4,643	101	364	16	31
Maryland	1,752	17,873	113	1,810	648	121
Massachusetts	5,066	24,287	128	3,431	1,836	159
Michigan	3,904	33,752	111	3,936	1,973	231
Minnesota	618	14,431	104	1,097	182	117
Mississippi	391	9,902	101	939	176	51
Missouri	496	19,301	95	1,262	173	171
Montana	16	2,965	90	166	-	34
Nebraska	88	5,093	95	396	28	28
Nevada	292	8,081	100	744	220	38
New Hampshire	156	4,010	103	301	49	30
New Jersey	9,253	35,069	149	6,487	4,582	115
New Mexico	190	5,446	93	414	84	27
New York[7]	8,256	40,874	130	7,035	4,135	200

CDC data for May 22, 2020, part 3 of 3

Provisional Death Counts for Co
cdc.gov/nchs/nvss/vsrr/COVID19/
Google

New Mexico	**190**	5,446	93	414	84	27
New York[7]	**8,256**	40,874	130	7,035	4,135	200
New York City	**17,002**	40,229	236	8,742	6,560	937
North Carolina	**222**	18,651	63	1,208	87	196
North Dakota	**24**	1,839	83	167	10	19
Ohio	**1,101**	35,529	90	2,327	469	246
Oklahoma	**214**	10,642	85	983	87	99
Oregon	**137**	10,748	95	578	52	61
Pennsylvania	**4,439**	39,622	92	3,735	1,699	183
Rhode Island	**304**	3,045	93	261	110	24
South Carolina	**339**	16,102	106	1,023	131	95
South Dakota	**34**	2,354	93	182	13	21
Tennessee	**246**	22,827	100	1,704	105	124
Texas	**962**	61,339	99	4,620	405	325
Utah	**70**	5,990	102	334	26	40
Vermont	**51**	1,866	104	123	12	14
Virginia	**962**	22,339	105	1,394	329	110
Washington	**766**	17,726	100	1,460	409	103
West Virginia	**50**	5,864	84	438	12	58
Wisconsin	**419**	17,109	105	958	67	148
Wyoming	**-**	1,393	103	104	-	-
Puerto Rico	**110**	7,274	86	1,026	58	47

CDC data for May 29, 2020, part 1 of 3

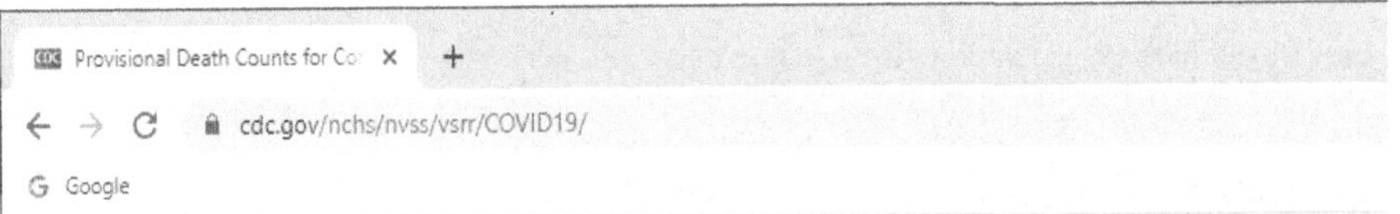

Table 2. Deaths involving coronavirus disease 2019 (COVID pneumonia, and influenza reported to NCHS by jurisdiction of United States. Week ending 2/1/2020 to 5/23/2020.*

Updated May 29, 2020

Jurisdiction of Occurrence	COVID-19 Deaths (U07.1)[1]	Deaths from All Causes	Percent of Expected Deaths[2]	Pneumonia Deaths (J12.0–J18.9)[3]
United States[6]	83,142	984,553	104	96,479
Alabama	511	16,937	96	1,109
Alaska	-	1,216	87	57
Arizona	631	21,199	105	1,601
Arkansas	95	10,285	96	703
California	2,963	91,713	101	8,260
Colorado	1,181	14,675	111	1,435
Connecticut	1,344	5,441	51	545
Delaware	258	3,063	100	248
District of Columbia	302	2,213	109	444
Florida	1,954	71,882	102	5,508
Georgia	1,346	27,525	98	2,069
Hawaii	16	3,755	97	242
Idaho	76	4,622	97	240

CDC data for May 29, 2020, part 2 of 3

Provisional Death Counts for Co

cdc.gov/nchs/nvss/vsrr/COVID19/

Google

Idaho	**76**	4,622	97	240
Illinois	**3,724**	39,807	112	4,424
Indiana	**1,656**	23,130	104	2,318
Iowa	**351**	9,908	98	717
Kansas	**180**	8,645	97	612
Kentucky	**329**	14,322	89	1,317
Louisiana	**1,943**	16,029	105	1,550
Maine	**77**	4,899	100	374
Maryland	**2,121**	19,227	115	2,002
Massachusetts	**5,647**	25,614	127	3,681
Michigan	**4,042**	36,254	111	4,119
Minnesota	**756**	15,354	104	1,182
Mississippi	**502**	10,908	104	1,054
Missouri	**547**	20,356	94	1,331
Montana	**16**	3,088	90	169
Nebraska	**116**	5,463	96	428
Nevada	**328**	8,603	100	794
New Hampshire	**198**	4,302	104	327
New Jersey	**10,702**	37,954	152	7,273
New Mexico	**234**	5,913	95	446
New York[7]	**9,015**	43,869	131	7,553
New York City	**17,880**	41,897	232	9,118
North Carolina	**328**	19,491	61	1,310

CDC data for May 29, 2020, part 3 of 3

Provisional Death Counts for Co ✕ +

cdc.gov/nchs/nvss/vsrr/COVID19/

Google

New Mexico	**234**	5,913	95	446	94
New York[7]	**9,015**	43,869	131	7,553	4,492
New York City	**17,880**	41,897	232	9,118	6,941
North Carolina	**328**	19,491	61	1,310	130
North Dakota	**32**	1,876	79	171	12
Ohio	**1,329**	38,444	93	2,533	563
Oklahoma	**224**	11,267	84	1,037	93
Oregon	**156**	11,461	94	609	59
Pennsylvania	**4,958**	42,623	93	4,022	1,884
Rhode Island	**428**	3,372	95	326	166
South Carolina	**363**	16,801	103	1,062	143
South Dakota	**44**	2,498	91	205	17
Tennessee	**280**	24,439	99	1,812	121
Texas	**1,209**	65,278	97	4,976	517
Utah	**84**	6,208	98	347	33
Vermont	**52**	1,967	102	124	12
Virginia	**1,168**	24,209	106	1,515	395
Washington	**918**	18,610	97	1,602	496
West Virginia	**60**	6,360	84	472	16
Wisconsin	**453**	18,095	102	998	73
Wyoming	**-**	1,486	98	108	-
Puerto Rico	**113**	8,360	86	1,148	60

CDC data for June 5, 2020, part 1 of 3

Provisional Death Counts for Co × +

cdc.gov/nchs/nvss/vsrr/COVID19/

Google

Table 2. Deaths involving coronavirus disease 2019 (COVID-19), pneumonia, and influenza repor NCHS by jurisdiction of occurrence, United States. Week ending 2/1/2020 to 5/30/2020.*

Updated June 5, 2020

Jurisdiction of Occurrence	COVID-19 Deaths (U07.1)[1]	Deaths from All Causes	Percent of Expected Deaths[2]	Pneumonia Deaths (J12.0–J18.9)[3]	Deaths with Pneumonia and COVID-19 (J12.0–J18.9 and U07.1)[3]	Influenza Deaths (J09–J11)[4]	Deaths with Pneumonia, Influenza, or COVID-19 U07.1 or J09–J18.9)[5]
United States[6]	**91,558**	1,053,901	105	103,367	39,953	6,372	160,417
Alabama	**601**	18,121	98	1,201	175	91	1,715
Alaska	-	1,301	88	61	-	-	71
Arizona	**734**	22,511	106	1,739	379	111	2,205
Arkansas	**105**	10,900	97	734	29	75	885
California	**3,581**	98,091	102	8,969	1,998	568	11,119
Colorado	**1,274**	15,497	111	1,509	665	93	2,206
Connecticut	**1,837**	7,424	66	774	424	63	2,249
Delaware	**339**	3,236	100	279	129	16	505
District of Columbia	**339**	2,410	113	487	339	-	495
Florida	**2,200**	76,465	103	5,872	1,146	304	7,223
Georgia	**1,533**	29,429	99	2,234	715	106	3,158
Hawaii	**16**	3,966	97	264	-	20	294
Idaho	**83**	4,952	99	253	25	25	336
Illinois	[illegible]	[illegible]	[illegible]	[illegible]	[illegible]	[illegible]	[illegible]

CDC data for June 5, 2020, part 2 of 3

Provisional Death Counts for Co

cdc.gov/nchs/nvss/vsrr/COVID19/

Google

Idaho	**83**	4,952	99	253	25	25	336
Illinois	**4,305**	42,609	114	4,825	2,214	176	7,089
Indiana	**1,868**	24,547	105	2,464	795	128	3,662
Iowa	**441**	10,549	99	779	124	84	1,180
Kansas	**194**	9,140	98	629	85	88	826
Kentucky	**370**	15,550	91	1,430	191	95	1,703
Louisiana	**2,149**	17,202	107	1,699	975	71	2,939
Maine	**86**	5,201	101	397	19	31	495
Maryland	**2,380**	20,414	116	2,147	871	123	3,763
Massachusetts	**6,288**	27,610	130	3,980	2,262	159	8,157
Michigan	**4,616**	38,962	114	4,495	2,326	236	7,017
Minnesota	**891**	16,303	105	1,262	264	118	2,006
Mississippi	**592**	11,673	105	1,149	274	51	1,518
Missouri	**643**	21,854	96	1,439	226	174	2,030
Montana	**16**	3,334	92	178	-	34	225
Nebraska	**149**	5,630	94	449	51	28	575
Nevada	**359**	9,128	100	838	263	39	973
New Hampshire	**226**	4,557	105	340	71	30	524
New Jersey	**11,345**	40,170	153	7,663	5,562	116	13,548
New Mexico	**257**	6,282	96	478	103	27	659
New York[7]	**9,549**	46,269	131	7,904	4,718	203	12,921
New York City	**18,375**	43,376	228	9,384	7,146	942	20,741
North Carolina	**462**	23,302	69	1,581	173	213	2,083

CDC data for June 5, 2020, part 3 of 3

Provisional Death Counts for Co ×

cdc.gov/nchs/nvss/vsrr/COVID19/

Google

New Jersey	**11,345**	40,170	153	7,663	5,562	116	13,548
New Mexico	**257**	6,282	96	478	103	27	659
New York[7]	**9,549**	46,269	131	7,904	4,718	203	12,921
New York City	**18,375**	43,376	228	9,384	7,146	942	20,741
North Carolina	**462**	23,302	69	1,581	173	213	2,083
North Dakota	**34**	1,988	79	174	12	19	215
Ohio	**1,577**	41,077	94	2,731	670	250	3,887
Oklahoma	**270**	12,656	90	1,148	108	105	1,410
Oregon	**163**	12,164	94	634	61	61	796
Pennsylvania	**5,557**	45,905	95	4,370	2,099	187	8,012
Rhode Island	**507**	3,668	99	370	200	25	702
South Carolina	**465**	18,200	105	1,166	185	98	1,543
South Dakota	**51**	2,638	92	212	19	26	270
Tennessee	**311**	25,838	99	1,907	131	125	2,212
Texas	**1,420**	69,672	98	5,344	612	332	6,481
Utah	**94**	6,741	101	369	37	40	466
Vermont	**52**	2,100	103	129	12	15	184
Virginia	**1,318**	25,629	106	1,597	439	111	2,585
Washington	**927**	20,194	100	1,669	503	109	2,197
West Virginia	**71**	6,709	84	496	22	58	603
Wisconsin	**519**	19,185	103	1,053	88	150	1,632
Wyoming	**11**	1,572	99	112	-	-	127
Puerto Rico	**123**	9,153	90	1,237	63	60	1,356

CDC data for June 12, 2020, part 1 of 3

Provisional Death Counts for Co

cdc.gov/nchs/nvss/vsrr/COVID19/

Google New Tab

Table 2. Deaths involving coronavirus disease 2019 (COVID-19), pneumonia, and influenza reported to NCHS by jurisdiction of occurrence, United States. Week ending 2/1/2020 to 6/6/2020.*

Updated June 12, 2020

Jurisdiction of Occurrence	All Deaths involving COVID-19 (U07.1)[1]	Deaths from All Causes	Percent of Expected Deaths[2]	Deaths involving Pneumonia, with or without COVID-19, excluding Influenza deaths (J12.0–J18.9)[3]	Deaths involving COVID-19 and Pneumonia, excluding Influenza (J12.0–J18.9 and U07.1)[3]	All Deaths involving Influenza, with or without COVID-19 or Pneumonia (J09–J11)[4]	Deaths involving Pneumonia, Influenza, or COVID-19 (U07.1 or J09–J18.9)[5]
United States[6]	**98,695**	1,116,797	104	109,291	42,863	6,401	170,596
Alabama	**678**	19,250	97	1,284	197	91	1,853
Alaska	-	1,368	87	65	-	-	75
Arizona	**858**	23,909	105	1,847	436	110	2,379
Arkansas	**125**	11,554	96	776	41	75	935
California	**4,007**	103,553	101	9,493	2,245	570	11,824
Colorado	**1,348**	16,373	109	1,573	695	95	2,316
Connecticut	**2,542**	8,472	72	953	576	64	2,982
Delaware	**378**	3,529	102	300	139	16	555
District of Columbia	**408**	2,615	115	560	407	-	569
Florida	**2,425**	80,711	101	6,227	1,265	305	7,685
Georgia	**1,682**	31,386	99	2,386	782	106	3,392
Hawaii	**16**	4,160	95	274	-	20	304

CDC data for June 12, 2020, part 2 of 3

Provisional Death Counts for Co ×

cdc.gov/nchs/nvss/vsrr/COVID19/

Google New Tab

Georgia	[illegible]	[illegible]	[illegible]	[illegible]	[illegible]	[illegible]	[illegible]
Hawaii	**16**	4,160	95	274	-	20	304
Idaho	**85**	5,241	97	262	25	25	347
Illinois	**4,932**	45,484	113	5,238	2,514	176	7,829
Indiana	**2,018**	25,904	103	2,587	851	129	3,880
Iowa	**534**	11,201	98	832	148	84	1,302
Kansas	**205**	9,586	96	656	88	89	862
Kentucky	**398**	16,462	91	1,513	203	95	1,802
Louisiana	**2,318**	18,230	107	1,833	1,064	71	3,153
Maine	**95**	5,467	98	409	21	31	514
Maryland	**2,685**	21,837	115	2,327	990	124	4,130
Massachusetts	**6,663**	28,909	127	4,174	2,394	161	8,596
Michigan	**4,838**	41,064	111	4,676	2,418	236	7,328
Minnesota	**1,037**	17,328	103	1,342	298	120	2,200
Mississippi	**696**	12,387	104	1,237	324	51	1,660
Missouri	**703**	23,315	95	1,502	237	175	2,143
Montana	**16**	3,564	93	189	-	34	236
Nebraska	**157**	6,077	95	471	54	28	602
Nevada	**392**	9,713	99	896	289	39	1,038
New Hampshire	**257**	4,802	102	356	80	30	562
New Jersey	**11,993**	42,211	151	8,093	5,895	116	14,293
New Mexico	**312**	6,748	96	521	128	29	734
New York[7]	**9,859**	48,444	128	8,166	4,859	205	13,354

CDC data for June 12, 2020, part 3 of 3

Provisional Death Counts for Co × +

cdc.gov/nchs/nvss/vsrr/COVID19/

Google New Tab

New Mexico	312	6,748	96	521	128	29	734
New York[7]	9,859	48,444	128	8,166	4,859	205	13,354
New York City	18,707	44,673	220	9,548	7,258	942	21,125
North Carolina	576	25,942	73	1,807	220	219	2,381
North Dakota	50	2,121	79	188	16	19	241
Ohio	1,806	43,657	94	2,928	756	251	4,228
Oklahoma	310	13,611	91	1,231	122	106	1,520
Oregon	174	12,918	94	660	65	61	829
Pennsylvania	5,887	48,746	93	4,571	2,197	187	8,445
Rhode Island	587	3,971	102	412	233	25	791
South Carolina	531	19,137	104	1,238	209	98	1,657
South Dakota	64	2,805	92	229	26	26	293
Tennessee	346	27,389	97	2,016	144	125	2,343
Texas	1,629	74,031	98	5,694	715	335	6,940
Utah	114	7,166	98	398	46	40	506
Vermont	53	2,243	102	138	12	15	194
Virginia	1,471	27,005	104	1,694	487	111	2,787
Washington	1,036	21,745	100	1,791	552	110	2,380
West Virginia	80	6,779	80	506	24	58	620
Wisconsin	593	20,330	102	1,111	100	150	1,752
Wyoming	13	1,674	99	113	-	-	130
Puerto Rico	130	9,644	89	1,289	68	61	1,411

[341] E Morath. How many US workers have lost jobs during coronavirus pandemic? There are several ways to count. Wall Street J. Jun 3 2020. https://www.wsj.com/articles/how-many-u-s-workers-have-lost-jobs-during-coronavirus-pandemic-there-are-several-ways-to-count-11591176601

[342] US Bureau of Labor Statistics. State employment and unemployment summary. https://www.bls.gov/news.release/laus.nr0.htm

[343] https://www.usatoday.com/storytelling/coronavirus-reopening-america-map/

344 https://www.cdc.gov/nchs/nvss/vsrr/COVID19/

cdc.gov/nchs/nvss/vsrr/COVID19/

Google New Tab

Table 1. Deaths involving coronavirus disease 2019 (COVID-19), pneumonia, and influenza reported to NCHS by week ending date, United States. Week ending 2/1/2020 to 6/20/2020.*

Updated June 26, 2020

Week ending date in which the death occurred	All Deaths involving COVID-19 (U07.1)[1]	Deaths from All Causes	Percent of Expected Deaths[2]	Deaths involving Pneumonia, with or without COVID-19, excluding Influenza deaths (J12.0–J18.9)[3]	Deaths involving COVID-19 and Pneumonia, excluding Influenza (U07.1 and J12.0–J18.9)[3]	All Deaths involving Influenza, with or without COVID-19 or Pneumonia (J09–J11), includes COVID-19 or Pneumonia[4]	Deaths involving Pneumonia, Influenza, or COVID-19 (U07.1 or J09–J18.9)[5]
Total Deaths	109,188	1,232,269	106	119,174	47,255	6,459	186,628
2/1/2020	1	58,179	98	3,766	0	477	4,244
2/8/2020	1	58,771	98	3,755	0	516	4,272
2/15/2020	0	57,904	98	3,770	0	549	4,319
2/22/2020	5	57,864	100	3,639	1	557	4,200
2/29/2020	5	58,250	101	3,762	3	638	4,402
3/7/2020	33	58,515	101	3,901	16	620	4,537
3/14/2020	52	57,428	101	3,883	27	611	4,518
3/21/2020	551	58,059	102	4,465	245	543	5,307
3/28/2020	3,052	62,067	111	6,049	1,376	439	8,114
4/4/2020	9,504	70,838	127	9,628	4,544	461	14,826
4/11/2020	15,698	77,492	140	11,712	7,030	468	20,510
4/18/2020	16,350	74,839	138	10,990	6,992	260	20,422
4/25/2020	14,103	70,998	132	9,710	6,038	143	17,822
5/2/2020	11,670	65,877	123	8,234	4,941	62	15,005
5/9/2020	10,747	63,528	121	7,494	4,551	46	13,727
5/16/2020	8,772	59,998	115	6,383	3,632	19	11,539
5/23/2020	6,666	56,162	108	5,404	2,793	20	9,295
5/30/2020	5,445	52,943	101	4,648	2,207	10	7,896

[345] https://medium.com/@JohnPospichal/questions-for-lockdown-apologists-32a9bbf2e247

[346] https://doi.org/10.1101/2020.04.24.20078717. https://www.medrxiv.org/content/10.1101/2020.04.24.20078717v1

[347] https://www.wsj.com/articles/do-lockdowns-save-many-lives-is-most-places-the-data-say-no-11587930911

[348] https://www.wsj.com/articles/how-many-u-s-workers-have-lost-jobs-during-coronavirus-pandemic-there-are-several-ways-to-count-11591176601

[349] https://www.bls.gov/news.release/laus.nr0.htm

[350] CDC. Weekly counts of deaths by jurisdiction and race and Hispanic origin. Mar 24 2021. https://data.cdc.gov/NCHS/Weekly-counts-of-deaths-by-jurisdiction-and-race-a/qfhf-uhaa

[351] Governing. State population by race, ethnicity data. From 2017 1-year American community survey estimates. US Census Bureau. https://www.governing.com/archive/state-minority-population-data-estimates.html

[352] G Briand. COVID-19 deaths: A look at US data. Mar 18 2021. PDMJ. https://pdmj.org/papers/Briand_look_at_US_data/

[353] The COVID Tracking Project. https://covidtracking.com/

[354] A McCann. States with the fewest coronavirus restrictions. Mar 2 2021. WalletHub. https://wallethub.com/edu/states-coronavirus-restrictions/73818

[355] Burbio's K-12 school opening tracker. Mar 31 2021. https://cai.burbio.com/school-opening-tracker/

[356] US Bureau of Labor Statistics. Mar 26 2021. https://www.bls.gov/news.release/laus.nr0.htm

[357] L Mineo. The main public health tool during 1918 pandemic? Social distancing. Mar 25 2021.The Harvard Gazette. https://news.harvard.edu/gazette/story/2021/03/harvard-experts-discuss-the-history-of-social-distancing/

[358] O Waxman. The surprisingly deep – and often troubling – history of 'social distancing.' Jun 30 2020. Time. https://time.com/5856800/social-distancing-history/

[359] C Wark, J Galliher. Emory Bogardus and the origins of the Social Distance Scale. Dec 2007. Am Sociologist. 38 (4). 383-395. https://www.researchgate.net/publication/226419827_Emory_Bogardus_and_the_Origins_of_the_Social_Distance_Scale#pfd

[360] USC Bogardus Papers, Nov 16 1970. https://www.researchgate.net/publication/226419827_Emory_Bogardus_and_the_Origins_of_the_Social_Distance_Scale#pfd

[361] E Hughes, C Johnson, et al. (Eds.) In *The Collected Papers of Robert E Park, Vol I, Race and Culture.* 1950. Glencoe, IL: The Free Press. https://catalogue.nla.gov.au/Record/1876301

[362] T Inglesby, J Nuzzo, et al. Disease mitigation measures in the control of pandemic influenza. 2006. Biosec Bioterr Biodefense Strategy. 4 (4). https://www.documentcloud.org/documents/6841076-2006-11-Disease-Mitigation-Measures-in-the.html

[363] J Aledorf, N Lurie, et al. Non-pharmaceutical public health interventions for pandemic influenza: an evaluation of the evidence base. Aug 15 2007. BMC Public Health. https://www.ncbi.nlm.nih.gov/pmc/articles/PMC2040158/

[364] World Health Organization Writing Group. Nonpharmaceutical public health interventions for pandemic influenza, national and community measures. 2006. Emerg Infec Dis. 12. 88-94. https://pubmed.ncbi.nlm.nih.gov/17697389/

[365] E Lipton, J Steinhauer. The untold story of the birth of social distancing. Apr 22 2020. New York Times. https://www.nytimes.com/2020/04/22/us/politics/social-distancing-coronavirus.html

[366] S Gottlieb. Where's the science behind CDC's 6-foot social-distance decree? Mar 21 2021. Wall Street J. https://www.wsj.com/articles/wheres-the-science-behind-cdcs-6-foot-social-distance-decree-11616358952

[367] D Chu, E Aki, et al. Physical distancing, face masks, and eye protection to prevent person-to person transmission of SARS-CoV-2 and COVID-19: a systematic review and meta-analysis. Jun 1 2020. The Lancet. 395 (10242). 1973-1987. https://www.thelancet.com/journals/lancet/article/PIIS0140-6736(20)31142-9/fulltext

[368] S Cao, Y Gan, et al. Post-lockdown SARS-CoV-2 nucleic acid screening in nearly ten million residents of Wuhan, China. Nov 20 2020. Nature Communications. 11. 5917 (2020). https://www.nature.com/articles/s41467-020-19802-w

[369] Z Madewell, Y Yang, et al. Household transmission of SARS-CoV-2. Dec 14 2020. JAMA. 3 (12) :e2031756 https://jamanetwork.com/journals/jamanetworkopen/fullarticle/2774102

[370] B Stadler. Coronavirus: Why everyone was wrong. Jul 1 2020. Medium. https://backtoreason.medium.com/coronavirus-why-everyone-was-wrong-fce6db5ba809

Masks: Not effective and not safe

[371] T Jefferson, M Jones, et al. Physical interventions to interrupt or reduce the spread of respiratory viruses. MedRxiv. 2020 Apr 7. https://www.medrxiv.org/content/10.1101/2020.03.30.20047217v2

[372] J Xiao, E Shiu, et al. Nonpharmaceutical measures for pandemic influenza in non-healthcare settings – personal protective and environmental measures. Centers for Disease Control. 26(5); 2020 May. https://wwwnc.cdc.gov/eid/article/26/5/19-0994_article

[373] J Brainard, N Jones, et al. Facemasks and similar barriers to prevent respiratory illness such as COVID19: A rapid systematic review. MedRxiv. 2020 Apr 1. https://www.medrxiv.org/content/10.1101/2020.04.01.20049528v1.full.pdf

[374] L Radonovich M Simberkoff, et al. N95 respirators vs medical masks for preventing influenza among health care personnel: a randomized clinic trial. JAMA. 2019 Sep 3. 322(9): 824-833. https://jamanetwork.com/journals/jama/fullarticle/2749214

[375] J Smith, C MacDougall. CMAJ. 2016 May 17. 188(8); 567-574. https://www.cmaj.ca/content/188/8/567

[376] F bin-Reza, V Lopez, et al. The use of masks and respirators to prevent transmission of influenza: a systematic review of the scientific evidence. 2012 Jul; 6(4): 257-267. https://www.ncbi.nlm.nih.gov/pmc/articles/PMC5779801/

[377] J Jacobs, S Ohde, et al. Use of surgical face masks to reduce the incidence of the common cold among health care workers in Japan: a randomized controlled trial. Am J Infect Control. 2009 Jun; 37(5): 417-419. https://pubmed.ncbi.nlm.nih.gov/19216002/

[378] M Viola, B Peterson, et al. Face coverings, aerosol dispersion and mitigation of virus transmission risk. https://arxiv.org/abs/2005.10720, https://arxiv.org/ftp/arxiv/papers/2005/2005.10720.pdf

[379] S Grinshpun, H Haruta, et al. Performance of an N95 filtering facepiece particular respirator and a surgical mask during human breathing: two pathways for particle penetration. J Occup Env Hygiene. 2009; 6(10):593-603. https://www.tandfonline.com/doi/pdf/10.1080/15459620903120086

[380] H Jung, J Kim, et al. Comparison of filtration efficiency and pressure drop in anti-yellow sand masks, quarantine masks, medical masks, general masks, and handkerchiefs. Aerosol Air Qual Res. 2013 Jun. 14:991-1002. https://aaqr.org/articles/aaqr-13-06-oa-0201.pdf

[381] C MacIntyre, H Seale, et al. A cluster randomized trial of cloth masks compared with medical masks in healthcare workers. BMJ Open. 2015; 5(4) https://bmjopen.bmj.com/content/5/4/e006577.long

[382] N95 masks explained. https://www.honeywell.com/en-us/newsroom/news/2020/03/n95-masks-explained

[383] V Offeddu, C Yung, et al. Effectiveness of masks and respirators against infections in healthcare workers: A systematic review and meta-analysis. Clin Inf Dis. 65(11), 2017 Dec 1; 1934-1942. https://academic.oup.com/cid/article/65/11/1934/4068747

[384] C MacIntyre, Q Wang, et al. A cluster randomized clinical trial comparing fit-tested and non-fit-tested N95 respirators to medical masks to prevent respiratory virus infection in health care workers. Influenza J. 2010 Dec 3. https://onlinelibrary.wiley.com/doi/epdf/10.1111/j.1750-2659.2011.00198.x?fbclid=IwAR3kRYVYDKb0aR-su9_me9_vY6a8KVR4HZ17J2A_80f_fXUABRQdhQlc8Wo

[385] M Walker. Study casts doubt on N95 masks for the public. MedPage Today. 2020 May 20. https://www.medpagetoday.com/infectiousdisease/publichealth/86601

[386] C MacIntyre, Q Wang, et al. A cluster randomized clinical trial comparing fit-tested and non-fit-tested N95 respirators to medical masks to prevent respiratory virus infection in health care workers. Influenza J. 2010 Dec 3. https://onlinelibrary.wiley.com/doi/epdf/10.1111/j.1750-2659.2011.00198.x?fbclid=IwAR3kRYVYDKb0aR-su9_me9_vY6a8KVR4HZ17J2A_80f_fXUABRQdhQlc8Wo

[387] N Shimasaki, A Okaue, et al. Comparison of the filter efficiency of medical nonwoven fabrics against three different microbe aerosols. Biocontrol Sci. 2018; 23(2). 61-69.
https://www.jstage.jst.go.jp/article/bio/23/2/23_61/_pdf/-char/en

[388] T Tunevall. Postoperative wound infections and surgical face masks: A controlled study. World J Surg. 1991 May; 15: 383-387.
https://link.springer.com/article/10.1007%2FBF01658736

[389] N Orr. Is a mask necessary in the operating theatre? Ann Royal Coll Surg Eng 1981: 63: 390-392.
https://www.ncbi.nlm.nih.gov/pmc/articles/PMC2493952/pdf/annrcse01509-0009.pdf

[390] N Mitchell, S Hunt. Surgical face masks in modern operating rooms – a costly and unnecessary ritual? J Hosp Infection. 18(3); 1991 Jul 1. 239-242.
https://www.journalofhospitalinfection.com/article/0195-6701(91)90148-2/pdf

[391] C DaZhou, P Sivathondan, et al. Unmasking the surgeons: the evidence base behind the use of facemasks in surgery. JR Soc Med. 2015 Jun; 108(6): 223-228.
https://www.ncbi.nlm.nih.gov/pmc/articles/PMC4480558/

[392] L Brosseau, M Sietsema. Commentary: Masks for all for Covid-19 not based on sound data. U Minn Ctr Inf Dis Res Pol. 2020 Apr 1.
https://www.cidrap.umn.edu/news-perspective/2020/04/commentary-masks-all-covid-19-not-based-sound-data

[393] N Leung, D Chu, et al. Respiratory virus shedding in exhaled breath and efficacy of face masks Nature Research. 2020 Mar 7. 26,676-680 (2020).
https://www.researchsquare.com/article/rs-16836/v1

[394] S Rengasamy, B Eimer, et al. Simple respiratory protection – evaluation of the filtration performance of cloth masks and common fabric materials against 20-1000 nm size particles. Ann Occup Hyg. 2010 Oct; 54(7): 789-798.
https://academic.oup.com/annweh/article/54/7/789/202744

[395] S Bae, M Kim, et al. Effectiveness of surgical and cotton masks in blocking SARS-CoV-2: A controlled comparison in 4 patients. Ann Int Med. 2020 Apr 6.
https://www.acpjournals.org/doi/10.7326/M20-1342

[396] S Rengasamy, B Eimer, et al. Simple respiratory protection – evaluation of the filtration performance of cloth masks and common fabric materials against 20-1000 nm size particles. Ann Occup Hyg. 2010 Oct; 54(7): 789-798.
https://academic.oup.com/annweh/article/54/7/789/202744

[397] C MacIntyre, H Seale, et al. A cluster randomized trial of cloth masks compared with medical masks in healthcare workers. BMJ Open. 2015; 5(4)
https://bmjopen.bmj.com/content/5/4/e006577.long

[398] W Kellogg. An experimental study of the efficacy of gauze face masks. Am J Pub Health. 1920. 34-42.
https://ajph.aphapublications.org/doi/pdf/10.2105/AJPH.10.1.34

[399] E Fischer, M Fischer, et al. Low-cost measurement of face mask efficacy for filtering expelled droplets during speech. Science Advances. Sep 2 2020. 6 (36).
https://advances.sciencemag.org/content/6/36/eabd3083?fbclid=IwAR0TPVlflF_sUEiSdad6oM1NVQGO5w2S7WfstCIKalJ15JJaKaDMzBkD5YY

[400] M Klompas, C Morris, et al. Universal masking in hospitals in the Covid-19 era. N Eng J Med. 2020; 382 e63.
https://www.nejm.org/doi/full/10.1056/NEJMp2006372

[401] E Person, C Lemercier et al. Effect of a surgical mask on six minute walking distance. Rev Mal Respir. 2018 Mar; 35(3):264-268.
https://pubmed.ncbi.nlm.nih.gov/29395560/

[402] B Chandrasekaran, S Fernandes. Exercise with facemask; are we handling a devil's sword – a physiological hypothesis. Med Hypothese. 2020 Jun 22. 144:110002.
https://pubmed.ncbi.nlm.nih.gov/32590322/

[403] P Shuang Ye Tong, A Sugam Kale, et al. Respiratory consequences of N95-type mask usage in pregnant healthcare workers – A controlled clinical study. Antimicrob Resist Infect Control. 2015 Nov 16; 4:48. https://pubmed.ncbi.nlm.nih.gov/26579222/

[404] T Kao, K Huang, et al. The physiological impact of wearing an N95 mask during hemodialysis as a precaution against SARS in patients with end-stage renal disease. J Formos Med Assoc. 2004 Aug; 103(8):624-628. https://pubmed.ncbi.nlm.nih.gov/15340662/

[405] F Blachere, W Lindsley et al. Assessment of influenza virus exposure and recovery from contaminated surgical masks and N95 respirators. J Viro Methods. 2018 Oct; 260:98-106. https://pubmed.ncbi.nlm.nih.gov/30029810/

[406] A Rule, O Apau, et al. Healthcare personnel exposure in an emergency department during influenza season. PLoS One. 2018 Aug 31; 13(8): e0203223. https://pubmed.ncbi.nlm.nih.gov/30169507/

[407] F Blachere, W Lindsley et al. Assessment of influenza virus exposure and recovery from contaminated surgical masks and N95 respirators. J Viro Methods. 2018 Oct; 260:98-106. https://pubmed.ncbi.nlm.nih.gov/30029810/

[408] A Chughtai, S Stelzer-Braid, et al. Contamination by respiratory viruses on our surface of medical masks used by hospital healthcare workers. BMC Infect Dis. 2019 Jun 3; 19(1): 491. https://pubmed.ncbi.nlm.nih.gov/31159777/

[409] L Zhiqing, C Yongyun, et al. J Orthop Translat. 2018 Jun 27; 14:57-62. https://pubmed.ncbi.nlm.nih.gov/30035033/

[410] C MacIntyre, H Seale, et al. A cluster randomized trial of cloth masks compared with medical masks in healthcare workers. BMJ Open. 2015; 5(4) https://bmjopen.bmj.com/content/5/4/e006577

[411] A Beder, U Buyukkocak, et al. Preliminary report on surgical mask induced deoxygenation during major surgery. Neurocirugia. 2008; 19: 121-126. http://scielo.isciii.es/pdf/neuro/v19n2/3.pdf

[412] D Lukashev, B Klebanov, et al. Cutting edge: Hypoxia-inducible factor 1-alpha and its activation-inducible short isoform negatively regulate functions of CD4+ and CD8+ T lymphocytes. J Immunol. 2006 Oct 15; 177(8) 4962-4965.
https://www.jimmunol.org/content/177/8/4962

[413] A Sant, A McMichael. Revealing the role of CD4+ T-cells in viral immunity. J Exper Med. 2012 Jun 30; 209(8):1391-1395.
https://europepmc.org/article/PMC/3420330

Masks and particulate inhalation

[414] C Huber. Masks are neither effective nor safe: A summary of the science. Jul 6 2020. Primary Doctor.
https://www.primarydoctor.org/masks-not-effect

[415] Occupational Safety and Health Administration (OSHA), US Department of Labor. Confined or enclosed spaces and other dangerous atmospheres.
https://www.osha.gov/SLTC/etools/shipyard/shiprepair/confinedspace/oxygendeficient.html

[416] S Sharma, B. Brown. Spirometry and respiratory muscle function during ascent to higher altitudes. Lung. Mar-Apr 2007. 185 (2): 113-21. doi: 10.1007/s00408-006-0108-y https://pubmed.ncbi.nlm.nih.gov/17393241/

[417] S Malik, I Singh. Ventilatory capacity among highland Bods: a possible adaptive mechanism at high altitude. Ann Hum Biol. Sep-Oct 1979. 6 (5) 471-6. doi: 10.1080/03014467900003851
https://pubmed.ncbi.nlm.nih.gov/533244/

[418] W Williams. Physiological response to alterations in [O2] and [CO2]: relevance to respiratory protective devices. J Int Soc Resp Protection. National Institute for Occupational Safety and Health (NIOSH). 27 (1): 27-51. 2010. https://www.isrp.com/the-isrp-journal/journal-public-abstracts/1154-vol-27-no-1-2010-pp-27-51-wiliams-open-access/file

[419] I Holmer, K Kuklane et al. Minute volumes and inspiratory flow rates during exhaustive treadmill walking using respirators. Ann Occup Hygiene. 51 (3): 327-335. Apr 2007. https://doi.org/10.1093/annhyg/mem004 https://academic.oup.com/annweh/article/51/3/327/139423

[420] H Kobayashi, S Kanoh, et al. Diffuse lung disease caused by cotton fibre inhalation but distinct from byssinosis. Thorax. Nov 2004. 59 (12). https://thorax.bmj.com/content/59/12/1095

[421] P Lai, D Christiani. Long-term respiratory health effects in textile workers. Curr Opin Pulm Med. Mar 2013. 19 (2): 152-157. doi: https://pubmed.ncbi.nlm.nih.gov/23361196/ https://www.ncbi.nlm.nih.gov/pmc/articles/PMC3725301/

[422] O Fadare, E Okoffo. Covid-19 face masks: A potential source of microplastic fibers in the environment. Sci Total Environ. Oct 1 2020. 737:140279. doi: 10.1016/j.scitotenv.2020.140279 https://www.ncbi.nlm.nih.gov/pmc/articles/PMC7297173/

[423] Ibid O Fadare, E Okoffo.

[424] J Cortez Pimentel, R Avila et al. Respiratory disease caused by synthetic fibers: a new occupational disease. Thorax. 1975. 30 (204): 205-19. https://www.ncbi.nlm.nih.gov/pmc/articles/PMC470268/pdf/thorax00140-0084.pdf

[425] Z Liu, D Yu, et al. Understanding the factors involved in determining the bioburdens of surgical masks. Ann Trans Med. Dec 2019. 7 (23). http://atm.amegroups.com/article/view/32465/html

[426] W Wuyts, C Agostini, et al. The pathogenesis of pulmonary fibrosis: a moving target. Eur Rep J. 2013 (41): 1207-1218. DOI: 10.1183/09031936.00073012 https://erj.ersjournals.com/content/41/5/1207

[427] G Oberdorster, E Oberdorster, et al. Nanotoxicology: An emerging discipline evolving from studies of ultrafine particles. Environ Health Perspect. Jul 2005. 113(7): 823-839. doi: 10.1289/ehp.7339 https://www.ncbi.nlm.nih.gov/pmc/articles/PMC1257642/

[428] C Scotton, R Chambers. Molecular targets in pulmonary fibrosis: the myofibroblast in focus. Chest. Oct 2007. 132 (4) 1311-21. doi: 10.1378/chest.06-2568. https://pubmed.ncbi.nlm.nih.gov/17934117/

[429] J Byrne, J Baugh. The significance of nanoparticles in particle-induced pulmonary fibrosis. McGill J Med. Jan 2008. 11 (1): 43-50. https://www.ncbi.nlm.nih.gov/pmc/articles/PMC2322933/

[430] D Bodian, H Howe. Experimental studies on intraneural spread of poliomyelitis virus. Bull Johns Hopkins Hops. 1941a; 69:248-267. https://www.cabdirect.org/cabdirect/abstract/19422700792

[431] International Commission on Radiological Protection. Human respiratory model for radiological protection. Ann ICRP. 1994. 24: 1-300. **The original of this article does not seem to be available. It was updated at this link:** https://www.researchgate.net/publication/5658235_Updating_the_ICRP_human_respiratory_tract_model

Masks and dysbiosis

[432] Y Huh, J Vosgerau, et al. Social defaults: Observed choices become choice defaults. J Consumer Research, Inc Chicago Journals. Aug 28 2014. 11:55 746-760. http://www.jstor.org/stable/10.1086/677315?origin=JSTOR-pdf

[433] Docs 4 Open Debate. Letter from medical doctors and health professionals to all Belgian authorities and all Belgian media. Sept 5 2020. https://docs4opendebate.be/en/open-letter/

[434] C Huber. Masks are neither effective nor safe. Primary Doctor. Jul 6 2020. https://www.primarydoctor.org/masks-not-effect

[435] C MacIntyre, H Seale, et al. A cluster randomized trial of cloth masks compared with medical masks in healthcare workers. BMJ Open. 2015; 5(4) https://bmjopen.bmj.com/content/5/4/e006577

[436] U Kelkar, B Gogate, et al. How effective are face masks in operation theatre? A time frame analysis and recommendations. Int J Inf Control. 2013. 9 (1). https://doi.org/10.3396/ijic.v9i1.10788 https://www.ijic.info/article/view/10788

[437] J Kwon, C Burnham, et al. Assessment of healthcare worker protocol deviations and self-contamination during personal protective equipment donning and doffing. Inf Control Hosp Epidemiol. Sep 2017. 38 (9): 1077-1083. https://dx.doi.org/10.1017%2Fice.2017.121. https://www.ncbi.nlm.nih.gov/pmc/articles/PMC6263164/

[438] N Orr. Is a mask necessary in the operating theatre? Ann Royal Coll Surg Eng. 1981. 63. 390-392. https://muchadoaboutcorona.ca/wp-content/uploads/2020/08/annrcse01509-0009.pdf

[439] N Mitchell, S Hunt. Surgical face masks in modern operating rooms – a costly and unnecessary ritual? J Hosp Inf. Jul 1991. 18 (3): 239-242. https://doi.org/10.1016/0195-6701(91)90148-2 https://www.sciencedirect.com/science/article/abs/pii/0195670191901482

[440] Michigan Medicine, University of Michigan. Estimating the size of a burn. https://www.uofmhealth.org/health-library/sig254759

[441] N Mitchell, S Hunt. Surgical face masks in modern operating rooms – a costly and unnecessary ritual? J Hosp Inf. Jul 1991. 18 (3): 239-242. https://doi.org/10.1016/0195-6701(91)90148-2 https://www.sciencedirect.com/science/article/abs/pii/0195670191901482

[442] H McClure, C Talboys, et al. Surgical face masks and downward dispersal of bacteria. Anaesthesia. 53 (7). Apr 6 2002. https://doi.org/10.1046/j.1365-2044.1998.435-az0528.x. https://associationofanaesthetists-publications.onlinelibrary.wiley.com/doi/full/10.1046/j.1365-2044.1998.435-az0528.x

[443] R Schweizer. Mask wiggling as a potential cause of wound contamination. Lancet. Nov 20 1976. 2 (7995). 1129-1130. doi: 10.1016/s0140-6736(76)91101-6 https://pubmed.ncbi.nlm.nih.gov/62960/

[444] New South Wales Government, National Centre for Immunisation Research and Surveillance. COVID-19 in schools – the experience in NSW. http://ncirs.org.au/sites/default/files/2020-04/NCIRS%20NSW%20Schools%20COVID_Summary_FINAL%20public_26%20April%202020.pdf

[445] C Felter, N Bussemaker. Which countries are requiring face masks? Council on Foreign Relations. Aug 4, 2020. https://www.cfr.org/in-brief/which-countries-are-requiring-face-masks

[446] Worldometers. https://www.worldometers.info/coronavirus/?%3D%3D

[447] R Channappanavar, S Perlman. Pathogenic human coronavirus infections: causes and consequences of cytokine storm and immunopathology. Semin Immunopathol. Jul 2017. 39 (5): 529-539. doi: 10.1007/s00281-017-0629-x. https://pubmed.ncbi.nlm.nih.gov/28466096/

[448] D Morens, J Taubenberger, et al. Predominant role of bacterial pneumonia as a cause of death in pandemic influenza: implications for pandemic influenza preparedness. J Inf Dis. Octo 1 2008. 198 (7). 962-970. https://doi.org/10.1086/591708. https://academic.oup.com/jid/article/198/7/962/2192118

[449] E Opie, F Blake, et al. The pathology and bacteriology of pneumonia following influenza. Chapter IV, Epidemic respiratory disease. The pneumonias and other infections of the respiratory tract accompanying influenza and measles. 1921, St. Louis. CV Mosby. 107-281.

[450] W Vaughan. Influenza: An epidemiologic study. Baltimore MD: Am J Hygiene. Monographic series. 1921. 1. 241.

[451] A Ciani. A pandemic of socialism. American Thinker. Aug 24, 2020. https://www.americanthinker.com/articles/2020/08/a_pandemic_of_socialism.html#ixzz6ZkgXX16k

[452] D Almond, B Mazumder. The 1918 influenza pandemic and subsequent health outcomes: An analysis of SIPP data. Am Econ Rev. May 2005. 95 (2): 258-262. doi: 10.1257/000282805774669943. https://pubmed.ncbi.nlm.nih.gov/29125265/

[453] A Prussin, E Garcia, et al. Total virus and bacteria concentrations in indoor and outdoor air. Environ Sci Technol Lett. 2015. 2 (4). 84-88. https://dx.doi.org/10.1021%2Facs.estlett.5b00050 https://www.ncbi.nlm.nih.gov/pmc/articles/PMC4515362/

[454] Blick. Your corona mask really is that gruesome. [article in German]. Sep 16, 2020. https://amp.blick.ch/wirtschaft/gebrauchte-exemplare-getestet-so-gruusig-ist-ihre-corona-maske-wirklich-id16096358.html?utm_source=twitter&utm_medium=social_user&utm_campaign=blick_amp

[455] L Zhiqing, C Yongyun. Surgical masks as source of bacterial contamination during operative procedures. J Ortho Translation. July 2018. 14. 57-62. https://doi.org/10.1016/j.jot.2018.06.002 https://www.sciencedirect.com/science/article/pii/S2214031X18300809

[456] P Luksamijarulkul, N Ajempradit, et al. Microbial contamination on used surgical masks among hospital personnel and microbial air quality in their working wards: A hospital in Bangkok. Oman Med J. Sept 2014. 29 (5). 346-350. https://dx.doi.org/10.5001%2Fomj.2014.92. https://www.ncbi.nlm.nih.gov/pmc/articles/PMC4202234/

[457] U Kelkar, B Gogate, et al. How effective are face masks in operation theatre? A time frame analysis and recommendations. Int J Inf Control. 2013. 9 (1). https://doi.org/10.3396/ijic.v9i1.10788 https://www.ijic.info/article/view/10788

[458] C MacIntyre, H Seale, et al. A cluster randomized trial of cloth masks compared with medical masks in healthcare workers. BMJ Open. 2015; 5(4) https://bmjopen.bmj.com/content/5/4/e006577

[459] J Xiao, E Shiu, et al. Nonpharmaceutical measures for pandemic influenza in non-healthcare settings – personal protective and environmental measures. Centers for Disease Control. 26(5); 2020 May. https://wwwnc.cdc.gov/eid/article/26/5/19-0994_article

[460] J Manley. Medical Doctor warns that "bacterial pneumonias are on the rise" from mask wearing. Oct 6 2020. https://www.globalresearch.ca/medical-doctor-warns-bacterial-pneumonias-rise-mask-wearing/5725848

[461] C Cichoracki. Health department investigating after high number of strep throat cases reported at Shepherd schools. ABC News. Oct 2 2020. https://www.abc12.com/app/2020/10/02/health-department-investigating-after-high-number-of-strep-throat-cases-at-shepherd-schools/?fbclid=IwAR2ECNvuIrMVGX_1adk_btUieta6sUPfCTu532-2UC2inKv6m9Hmb8Ey3W4

---

[462] US Centers for Disease Control. Coronavirus disease 2019 (COVID-19). Sep 10 2020 update. https://www.cdc.gov/coronavirus/2019-ncov/hcp/planning-scenarios.html#table-1

[463] R Schnirman, N Nur et al. A case of legionella pneumonia caused by home use of continuous positive airway pressure. SAGE Open Med Case Rep. 2017; 5: 2050313X17744981. doi:10.1177/2050313X1774498 https://journals.sagepub.com/doi/10.1177/2050313X17744981

[464] F Scannapieco. Role of oral bacteria in respiratory infection. J Periodontol. Jul 1999. 70 (7): 793-802. doi: 10.1902/jop.1999.70.7.793. https://pubmed.ncbi.nlm.nih.gov/10440642/

[465] O Ortega, P Clave. Oral hygiene, aspiration and aspiration pneumonia: From pathophysiology to therapeutic strategies. Curr Phys Med Rehabil Rep. Oct 2013. 1:292-295. DOI 10.1007/s40141-013-0032-z.

[466] R Ramondi. Interview with FOX News. 'Mask mouth': Dentists coin new term for smelly side effect of wearing a mask. Aug 7 2020. https://www.foxnews.com/health/mask-mouth-dentists-new-term

[467] I Holmer, K Kuklane et al. Minute volumes and inspiratory flow rates during exhaustive treadmill walking using respirators. Ann Occup Hygiene. 51 (3): 327-335. Apr 2007. https://doi.org/10.1093/annhyg/mem004 https://academic.oup.com/annweh/article/51/3/327/139423

[468] OA Khair, RJ Davies, et al. Bacterial-induced release of inflammatory mediators by bronchial epithelial cells. Eur Resp J. 1996(9): 1913-1922. https://erj.ersjournals.com/content/9/9/1913

[469] F Scannapieco, B Wang, et al. Oral bacteria and respiratory infection: Effects on respiratory pathogen adhesion and epithelial cell proinflammatory cytokine production. Ann Periodontol. Dec 1, 2001. https://doi.org/10.1902/annals.2001.6.1.78 https://aap.onlinelibrary.wiley.com/doi/abs/10.1902/annals.2001.6.1.78

[470] J Patel, V Sampson. The role of oral bacteria in COVID-19. Lancet. https://doi.org/10.1016/S2666-5247(20)30057-4. https://www.thelancet.com/journals/lanmic/article/PIIS2666-5247(20)30057-4/fulltext

[471] A Azarpazhooh, JL Leake. Systematic review of the association between respiratory diseases and oral health. J Periodontol. 2006 (77): 1465-1482. https://pubmed.ncbi.nlm.nih.gov/16945022/

[472] P Sjogren, E Nilsson, et al. A systematic review of the preventive effect of oral hygiene on pneumonia and respiratory tract infection in elderly people in hospitals and nursing homes: effect estimates and methodological quality of randomized controlled trials. J Am Geriatr Soc. 2008 (56): 2124-2130. https://pubmed.ncbi.nlm.nih.gov/18795989/

[473] D Manger, M Walshaw, et al. Evidence summary: The relationship between oral health and pulmonary disease. Br Dent J. Apr 7 2017. 222 (7): 527-533. doi: 10.1038/sj.bdj.2017.315 https://pubmed.ncbi.nlm.nih.gov/28387268/

[474] A Stacy, D Fleming et al. A commensal bacterium promotes virulence of an opportunistic pathogen via cross-respiration. Am Soc for Microbiol. 7 (3) e00782-16. doi:10.1128/mBio.00782-16 https://mbio.asm.org/content/7/3/e00782-16/article-info

[475] K Todar. The Normal Bacterial Flora of Humans. Online Textbook of Bacteriology. 2020. http://www.textbookofbacteriology.net/normalflora_3.html

[476] R Glaser, W Thomas, et al. The incidence and pathogenesis of myocarditis in rabbits after group A streptococcal pharyngeal infections. J Exp Med. Jan 1 1956.. 103 (1): 173-188. doi: 10.1084/jem.103.1.173. https://pubmed.ncbi.nlm.nih.gov/13278463/

[477] J Patel, V Sampson. The role of oral bacteria in COVID-19. Lancet. https://doi.org/10.1016/S2666-5247(20)30057-4. https://www.thelancet.com/journals/lanmic/article/PIIS2666-5247(20)30057-4/fulltext

[478] A Ramesh, S Varghese, et al. Chronic obstructive pulmonary disease and periodontitis – Unwinding their linking mechanisms. Sept 2015. J Oral Biosci. 58 (1). https://www.researchgate.net/publication/283116707_Chronic_obstructive_pulmonary_disease_and_periodontitis_-_Unwinding_their_linking_mechanisms

[479] P Heikkila, A But, et al. Periodontitis and cancer mortality: Register-based cohort study of 68,273 adults in 10-year follow-up. Cancer Epidem. Int J Cancer. 142 (11). Jan 11 2018. https://doi.org/10.1002/ijc.31254 https://onlinelibrary.wiley.com/doi/full/10.1002/ijc.31254

[480] N Babu, A Gomes. Systemic manifestations of oral diseases. J Oral Maxillofac Pathol. 15 (2); May-Aug 2011. https://dx.doi.org/10.4103%2F0973-029X.84477 https://www.ncbi.nlm.nih.gov/pmc/articles/PMC3329699/

[481] C Bingham, M Moni. Periodontal disease and rheumatoid arthritis: the evidence accumulates for complex pathobiologic interactions. Curr Opin Rheumatol. Jul 8 2015. https://dx.doi.org/10.1097%2FBOR.0b013e32835fb8ec https://www.ncbi.nlm.nih.gov/pmc/articles/PMC4495574/

[482] B Feldman. The oral microbiome and its links to autoimmunity. The Doctor Weighs In. Aug 26, 2018. https://thedoctorweighsin.com/oral-microbiome-links-autoimmunity/

[483] US Centers for Diseases Control. Erythromycin-resistant Group A Streptococcus. https://www.cdc.gov/drugresistance/pdf/threats-report/gas-508.pdf

[484] T Dileepan, E Smith, et al. Group A Streptococcus intranasal infection promotes CNS infiltration by streptococcal-specific Th17 cells. J Clin Invest. Jan 2016. 126 (1): 303-317. doi: 10.1172/JCI80792
https://pubmed.ncbi.nlm.nih.gov/26657857/

[485] Mayo Clinic. Staph Infections. [Article is now partially censored.]
https://www.mayoclinic.org/diseases-conditions/staph-infections/symptoms-causes/syc-20356221

[486] J Terrasse, J Lere, et al. Septicèmie, ostéomyelite, percardite suppurée a staphylocoques; guerison par la pénicilline intraveineuse, intramusculaire, intrapéricardique. [Article in French]. Bull Mem So Med Hop Paris, 1945. 61 (26-31): 400-402.
https://pubmed.ncbi.nlm.nih.gov/21021328/

[487] R Rubin, R Moellering. Clinical, microbiologic and therapeutic aspects of purulent pericarditis. Am J Med. Jul 1975. 59 (1): 68-78. doi: 10.1016/0002-9343(75)90323-x.
https://pubmed.ncbi.nlm.nih.gov/1138554/

[488] A Majid, A Omar. Diagnosis and management of purulent pericarditis. Experience with pericardiectomy. J Thorac Cardiovasc Surg. Sept 1991. 102 (3): 413-417.
https://pubmed.ncbi.nlm.nih.gov/1881180/

[489] S Pankuweit, A Ristic, et al. Bacterial pericarditis: diagnosis and management. Am J Cardiovasc Drugs. 2005. 5 (2): 103-112. doi: 10.2165/00129784-200505020-00004.
https://pubmed.ncbi.nlm.nih.gov/15725041/

[490] R Taib, D Penny. Infective Endocarditis. In Paediatric Cardiology. (Third Edition). 2010.
https://www.sciencedirect.com/book/9780702030642/paediatric-cardiology

[491] G Chhatwal, R Graham. Streptococcal diseases. In International Encyclopedia of Public Health (Second Edition). 2017. https://www.sciencedirect.com/referencework/9780128037089/international-encyclopedia-of-public-health

[492] A DeSoyza, S Alberti. Bronchiectasis and aspergillosis: How are they linked? Med Mycol Jan 1 2017. 55 (1): 69-81. doi: 10.1093/mmy/myw109. https://pubmed.ncbi.nlm.nih.gov/27794529/

[493] D Shah, S Jackman, et al. Effect of gliotoxin on human polymorphonuclear neutrophils. Infect Dis Obstet Gynecol. 1998. 6 (4). 168-175. https://dx.doi.org/10.1002%2F(SICI)1098-0997(1998)6%3A4%3C168%3A%3AAID-IDOG6%3E3.0.CO%3B2-Z https://www.ncbi.nlm.nih.gov/pmc/articles/PMC1784797/

Masks and physiological changes

[494] T Jacobson, J Kler, et al. Direct human health risks of increased atmospheric carbon dioxide. Nat Sustain. 2019. 2 (8). 691-701. https://www.nature.com/articles/s41893-019-0323-1

[495] D Sin, S Man, et al. Arterial carbon dioxide tension on admission as a marker of in-hospital mortality in community-acquired pneumonia. Am J Med. Feb 1 2005. 118 (2). 145-150. https://doi.org/10.1016/j.amjmed.2004.10.014 https://www.amjmed.com/article/S0002-9343(04)00680-1/fulltext

[496] P Murtagh, V Giubergia, et al. Lower respiratory infections by adenovirus in children. Clinical features and risk factors for bronchiolitis obliterans and mortality. Ped Pulm. 44. 450-456. https://doi.org/10.1002/ppul.20984 https://www.nature.com/articles/s41598-018-32008-x#ref-CR10

[497] N Nin, A Muriel et al. Severe hypercapnia and outcome of mechanically ventilated patients with moderate or severe acute respiratory distress syndrome. Int Care Med 43. 200-208. https://www.ncbi.nlm.nih.gov/pmc/articles/PMC5630225/

[498] K Moser, E Shibel, et al. Acute respiratory failure in obstructive lung disease. JAMA. Aug 13 1973. 225. 705-707. https://jamanetwork.com/journals/jama/article-abstract/349944

[499] B Chandrasekaran, S Fernandes. Exercise with facemask; Are we handling a devil's sword? – A physiological hypothesis. Nov 2020. 144 (110002). doi: 10.1016/j.mehy.2020.110002 https://www.ncbi.nlm.nih.gov/pmc/articles/PMC7306735/#b0135

[500] M Joyner, D Casey. Regulation of increased blood flow (hyperemia) to muscles during exercise: a hierarchy of competing physiological needs. Physiol Rev. Apr 2015. 95 (2). 549-601. doi: 10.1152/physrev.00035.2013. https://pubmed.ncbi.nlm.nih.gov/25834232/

[501] Carbon Dioxide Health Hazard Information Sheet. Food Safety Inspection Service, US Department of Agriculture. https://www.fsis.usda.gov/wps/wcm/connect/bf97edac-77be-4442-aea4-9d2615f376e0/Carbon-Dioxide.pdf?MOD=AJPERES

[502] Z Zhaoshi. Potential risks when some special people wear masks. No. 1 Dept of Neurology, The Third Hospital of Jilin University. Apr 18 2020. https://jamanetwork.com/journals/jama/fullarticle/2764955

[503] Carbon Dioxide Health Hazard Information Sheet. Food Safety Inspection Service, US Department of Agriculture. https://www.fsis.usda.gov/wps/wcm/connect/bf97edac-77be-4442-aea4-9d2615f376e0/Carbon-Dioxide.pdf?MOD=AJPERES

[504] Occupational Chemical Database: Carbon Dioxide. US Department of Labor, Occupational Safety and Health Administration. https://www.osha.gov/chemicaldata/chemResult.html?RecNo=183

[505] Carbon Dioxide Health Hazard Information Sheet. Food Safety Inspection Service, US Department of Agriculture. https://www.fsis.usda.gov/wps/wcm/connect/bf97edac-77be-4442-aea4-9d2615f376e0/Carbon-Dioxide.pdf?MOD=AJPERES

[506] Acid-base physiology, 4.4 Respiratory acidosis-Metabolic effects. https://www.anaesthesiamcq.com/AcidBaseBook/ab4_4.php

[507] J Williams, J Krah, et al. The physiological burden of prolonged PPE use on healthcare workers during long shifts. US Centers for Disease Control and Prevention. Jun 10 2020. https://blogs.cdc.gov/niosh-science-blog/2020/06/10/ppe-burden/

[508] R Roberge, A Coca, et al. Physiological impact of the N95 filtering facepiece respirator on healthcare workers. Respir Care. May 2010. 55 (5). 569-577. https://pubmed.ncbi.nlm.nih.gov/20420727/

[509] M Shigemura, e Lecuona et al. Effects of hypercapnia on the lung. J Physiol. Jan3 2017. 595 (8). https://doi.org/10.1113/JP273781 https://physoc.onlinelibrary.wiley.com/doi/full/10.1113/JP273781

[510] C Vohwinkel, E Lecuona et al. Elevated CO(2) levels cause mitochondrial dysfunction and impair cell proliferation. J Biol Chem. Oct 28 2011. 286 (43). 37067-76. doi: 10.1074/jbc.M111.290056. https://pubmed.ncbi.nlm.nih.gov/21903582/

[511] C Kempeneers, C Seaton, et al. Ciliary functional analysis: beating a path towards standardization. Pediatr Pulmonol. Oct 2019. 54 (10). 1627-1638. https://doi.org/10.1002/ppul.24439 https://pubmed.ncbi.nlm.nih.gov/31313529/

[512] E Laserna, O Sibila, et al. Hypocapnia and hypercapnia are predictors for ICU admission and mortality in hospitalized patients with community-acquired pneumonia. Chest. Nove 2012. 142 (5): 1193-1199. doi: 10.1378/chest.12-0576 https://pubmed.ncbi.nlm.nih.gov/22677348/

[513] A Lardner. The effects of extracellular pH on immune function. J Leukoc Biol. Apr 2001. 69 (4). 522-30 https://pubmed.ncbi.nlm.nih.gov/11310837/

[514] C Lang, P Dong, et al. Effect of CO2 on LPS-induced cytokine responses in rats alveolar macrophages. Am J Physiol Lung Cell Mol Physiol. Jul 2005. 289 (1). L96-L103. doi: 10.1152/ajplung.00394.2004 https://pubmed.ncbi.nlm.nih.gov/15778246/

[515] S Casalino-Matsuda, N Wang, et al. Hypercapnia alters expression of immune response, nucleosome assembly and lipid metabolism genes in differentiated human bronchial epithelial cells. Sep 10 2018. Sci Rep. 13508. https://www.nature.com/articles/s41598-018-32008-x

[516] D O'Croinin, et al. Sustained hypercapnic acidosis during pulmonary infection increases bacterial load and worsens lung injury. Crit Care Med. 36. 2128-2135. https://doi.org/10.1097/CCM.0b013e31817d1b59 https://pubmed.ncbi.nlm.nih.gov/18552698/

[517] B Borovoy, C Huber, Maria Crisler. Masks, false safety and real dangers, Part 2: Microbial challenges from masks. Oct 2020. https://PDMJ.org

[518] D Morens, J Taubenberger, et al. Predominant role of bacterial pneumonia as a cause of death in pandemic influenza: implications for pandemic influenza preparedness. J Inf Dis. Octo 1 2008. 198 (7). 962-970. https://doi.org/10.1086/591708. https://academic.oup.com/jid/article/198/7/962/2192118

[519] J Williams, J Cichowitz, et al. The physiological burden of prolonged PPE use on healthcare workers during long shifts. US Centers for Disease Control (CDC) National Institute of Occupational Safety and Health (NIOSH) Science Blog. Jun 10 2020. https://blogs.cdc.gov/niosh-science-blog/2020/06/10/ppe-burden/

[520] D Harmening. Clinical Hematology and Fundamentals of Hemostasis, 4th ed. Davis Company. 2002. 349.

[521] L Costanzo. Physiology. W B Saunders Company. 1998. 286-287.

[522] A Yartsev. Pharmacology of carbon dioxide. Deranged Physiology. https://derangedphysiology.com/main/cicm-primary-exam/required-reading/respiratory-system/Chapter%20311/pharmacology-carbon-dioxide

[523] A Voulgaris, O Marrone, et al. Chronic kidney disease in patients with obstructive sleep apnea. A narrative review. Sleep Med Rev. 2019. 10 (47). 74-89. https://pubmed.ncbi.nlm.nih.gov/31376590/

[524] Medicine Libre Texts. 6.4: Metabolic effects. Aug 13 2020. https://med.libretexts.org/Bookshelves/Anatomy_and_Physiology/Book%3A_Acid-base_Physiology_(Brandis)/06%3A_Respiratory_Acidosis/6.04%3A_Metabolic_Effects

[525] C Smith, J Whitelaw, et al. Carbon dioxide regreathing in respiratory protective devices: influence of speech and wor rate in full-face masks. Ergonomics. 2013. 56 (5): 781-790. https://pubmed.ncbi.nlm.nih.gov/23514282/

[526] D Stevens, B Jackson, et al. The impact of obstructive sleep apnoea on balance, gait and falls risk: a narrative review of the literature. J Gerontol A Biol Sci Med Sci. Feb 2020. 10glaa014. Online ahead of print. https://pubmed.ncbi.nlm.nih.gov/32039438/

[527] E Lim, R Seet, etal. Headaches and the N-95 face-mask amongst healthcare providers. Acta Neurol Scand Mar 2006. 113 (3). 199-202. doi: 10.1111/j.1600-0404.2005.00560.x https://pubmed.ncbi.nlm.nih.gov/16441251/

[528] N Fabregas, J Fernández-Candil. Hypercapnia. Dec 2016. In book Complications in Neuroanesthesia. 157-168. https://doi.org/10.1016/B978-0-12-804075-1.00020-1 https://www.sciencedirect.com/science/article/pii/B9780128040751000201?via%3Dihub

[529] J Sayers, R Smith, et al. Effects of carbon dioxide on mental performance. J Appl Physiol. Jul 1985. 63 (1). 25-30. doi: 10.1152/jappl.1987.63.1.25 https://pubmed.ncbi.nlm.nih.gov/3114218/

[530] U Satish, M Mendell, et al. Is CO2 an indoor pollutant? Direct effects of low-to-moderate CO2 concentrations on human decision-making performance. Environ Health Perspect. Dec 2012. 120 (12). 1671-1677. https://dx.doi.org/10.1289%2Fehp.1104789 https://www.ncbi.nlm.nih.gov/pmc/articles/PMC3548274/

[531] Y Yang, C Sun, et al. The effect of moderately increased CO2 concentration on perception of coherent motion. Aviat Space Environ Med. Mar 1997. 68 (3). 187-191. https://pubmed.ncbi.nlm.nih.gov/9056025/

[532] K Azuma, N Kagi, et al. Effects of low-level inhalation exposure to carbon dioxide in indoor environments: A short review on human health and psychomotor performance. Environ Int. Dec 2018. 121 (Pt1). 51-56. doi: 10.1016/j.envint.2018.08.059 https://pubmed.ncbi.nlm.nih.gov/30172928/

[533] A Beder, U Buyukkocak, et al. Preliminary report on surgical mask induced deoxygenation during major surgery. Neurocirugia 2008. 19. 121-126. http://scielo.isciii.es/pdf/neuro/v19n2/3.pdf

[534] T Kao, K Huang, et al. The physiological impact of wearing an N95 mask during hemodialysis as a precaution against SARS in patients with end-stage renal disease. J Formos Med Assoc. Aug 2004. 103 (8). 624-628. https://pubmed.ncbi.nlm.nih.gov/15340662/

[535] Bureau of Labor Statistics. News Release. USDL-11-1247. National Census of Fatal Occupational Injuries in 2010. Preliminary Results. Aug 25 2011. https://scholar.google.com/scholar?cluster=5019350129886890079&hl=en&as_sdt=805&sciodt=0,3

[536] D Spelce, R McKay, et al. Respiratory protection for oxygen deficient atmospheres. J Int Soc Respir Prot. 2016. 33 (2). https://www.ncbi.nlm.nih.gov/pmc/articles/PMC7183576/

[537] K Fedor. Noninvasive respiratory support in infants and children. Respiratory Care. Jun 2017. Vol 62 (6). 699-717. doi: 10.4187/respcare.05244 https://pubmed.ncbi.nlm.nih.gov/28546373/

[538] J Weinstein, J Smith. Pediatric BIPAP. J Emer Med Svcs. Sep 19 2019. https://www.jems.com/2019/09/19/pediatric-bipap/

[539] US Department of Labor, Occupational Safety & Health Administration. Confined or enclosed spaces and other dangerous atmospheres >> Oxygen deficient or oxygen enriched atmospheres. https://www.osha.gov/SLTC/etools/shipyard/shiprepair/confinedspace/oxygendeficient.html

[540] Z Zhaoshi. Potential risks when some special people wear masks. No. 1 Dept of Neurology, The Third Hospital of Jilin University. Apr 18 2020. https://jamanetwork.com/journals/jama/fullarticle/2764955

[541] C Luther. OSHA oxygen concentration standards. Sep 15 2020. https://work.chron.com/osha-oxygen-concentration-standards-15047.html

[542] D Spelce, R McKay, et al. Respiratory protection for oxygen deficient atmospheres. J Int Soc Respir Prot. 2016. 33 (2). https://www.ncbi.nlm.nih.gov/pmc/articles/PMC7183576/

[543] J Henry. Clinical Diagnosis and Management by Laboratory Methods. 19th ed. WB Saunders Co. © 1996. P. 86.

[544] T Carbonell, R Rama. Respiratory hypoxia and oxidative stress in the brain.Is the endogenous erythropoietin an antioxidant? Current Chem Biol. 2009. 3 (3). https://doi.org/10.2174/2212796810903030238 https://www.eurekaselect.com/93407/article/respiratory-hypoxia-and-oxidative-stress-brain-endogenous-erythropoietin-antioxidant

[545] K Blomgren, H Hagberg. Free radicals, mitochondria and hypoxia-ischemia in the developing brain. Free radic Biol Med. Feb 1 2006. 40 (3). 388-397. https://pubmed.ncbi.nlm.nih.gov/16443153/

[546] G Padhy, A Gangwar, et al. Plasma kallikrein-bradykinin pathway promotes circulatory nitric oxide metabolite availability during hypoxia. Nitric Oxide. Vol 55-56. May-June 2016. 36-44. https://www.sciencedirect.com/science/article/abs/pii/S1089860316300155

[547] J Greenwod. Mechanisms of blood-brain barrier breakdown. Neuroradiology. 1991. 33 (2): 95-100. doi: 10.1007/BF00588242. https://pubmed.ncbi.nlm.nih.gov/2046916/

[548] M Griesz-Brisson. Interview. Technocracy News. https://www.technocracy.news/german-neurologist-on-face-masks-oxygen-deprivation-causes-permanent-neurological-damage/

[549] C St. Croix, B Morgan, et al. Fatiguing inspiratory muscle work causes reflex sympathetic activation in humans. J Physiol. Dec 1 2000. 529 Pt 2 (Pt 2). 493-504. doi: 10.1111/j.1469-7793.2000.00493.x. https://pubmed.ncbi.nlm.nih.gov/11101657/

[550] V Melnikov, V Divert, et al. Baseline values of cardiovascular and respiratory parameters predict response to acute hypoxia in young healthy men. Physiol Res. 2017. 66 (3). 467-479. https://pubmed.ncbi.nlm.nih.gov/28248531/

[551] J Crawford, T Isbell, et al. Hypoxia, red blood cells, and nitrite regulate NO-dependent hypoxic vasodilation. Blood. Jan 15 2006. 107 (2). 566-574. https://dx.doi.org/10.1182%2Fblood-2005-07-2668 https://www.ncbi.nlm.nih.gov/pmc/articles/PMC1895612/

[552] J Henry. Clinical Diagnosis and Management by Laboratory Methods. 19th ed. WB Saunders Co. © 1996. P. 599.

[553] MedGen. Erythroid hyperplasia. https://www.ncbi.nlm.nih.gov/medgen/4536#rdis_1634824

[554] D Harmening. Clinical Hematology and Fundamentals of Hemostasis., 4th ed. Davis Company. 2002. 348-349.

[555] E Cummins, D Crean. Hypoxia and inflammatory bowel disease. Microbes and Infection. 19 (3). March 2017. 210-221. https://www.sciencedirect.com/science/article/abs/pii/S1286457916301319?via%3Dihub

[556] N Zeitouni, S Chotikatum, et al. The impact of hypoxia on intestinal epithelial cell functions: consequences for invasion by bacterial pathogens. Mol Cell Ped. 2016. 14. https://doi.org/10.1186/s40348-016-0041-y https://molcellped.springeropen.com/articles/10.1186/s40348-016-0041-y

[557] W Zhu. Should, and how can, exercise be done during a coronavirus outbreak? An interview with Dr. Jeffrey A Woods. J Sport Health Sci. Mar 2020. 9 (2). 105-107. doi: 10.1016/j.jshs.2020.01.005. https://pubmed.ncbi.nlm.nih.gov/32099717/

[558] M Hogan, R Cox, et al. Lactate accumulation during incremental exercise with varied inspired oxygen fractions. J Appl Physiol Respir Environ Exerc Physiol. Oct 1983. 55 (4). 1134-1140. doi: 10.1152/jappl.1983.55.4.1134 https://pubmed.ncbi.nlm.nih.gov/6629944/

[559] O Warburg. On the origin of cancer cells. Science. Feb 24 1956. 123 (3191). DOI:10.1126/science.123.3191.309. https://science.sciencemag.org/content/123/3191/309

[560] O Warburg. On the origin of cancer cells. Science. Feb 24 1956. 123 (3191). https://www.jstor.org/stable/1750066?seq=1

[561] A Chambers, S Matosevic. Immunometabolic dysfunction of natural killer cells mediated by the hypoxia-CD73 axis in solid tumors. Front Mol Biosci. 2019. 6 (60). Jul 24 2019. https://dx.doi.org/10.3389%2Ffmolb.2019.00060 https://www.ncbi.nlm.nih.gov/pmc/articles/PMC6668567/

[562] G Crittenden. Is your mask giving you lung cancer? Oct 21 2020. https://neverb4.net/is-your-mask-giving-you-lung-cancer/

[563] M Chua, W Cheng, et al. Face masks in the new COVID-19 normal: materials, testing and perspectives. Research (Wash DC) Aug 7 2020. https://dx.doi.org/10.34133%2F2020%2F7286735 https://www.ncbi.nlm.nih.gov/pmc/articles/PMC7429109/

[564] Solvay. Material for Covid-19 PPE and medical equipment: N-95 masks. https://www.solvay.com/en/chemical-categories/specialty-polymers/healthcare/medical-equipment-emergency-production/n95-masks

[565] M Chua, W Cheng, et al. Face masks in the new COVID-19 normal: materials, testing and perspectives. Research (Wash DC) Aug 7 2020. https://dx.doi.org/10.34133%2F2020%2F7286735 https://www.ncbi.nlm.nih.gov/pmc/articles/PMC7429109/

[566] P Pierozan, F Jemeren, et al. Perfluorooctanoic acid (PFOA) exposure promotes proliferation, migration and invasion potential in human breast epithelial cells. Arch Toxicol. 2018. (92 (5). 1729-1739. Mar 3 2018. https://dx.doi.org/10.1007%2Fs00204-018-2181-4 https://www.ncbi.nlm.nih.gov/pmc/articles/PMC5962621/

[567] K Steenland, T Fletcher, et al. Epidemiologic evidence on the health effects of perfluorooctanoic acid (PFOA). Environ Health Perspect. Aug 2010. 118 (8): 1100-1108. https://dx.doi.org/10.1289%2Fehp.0901827 https://www.ncbi.nlm.nih.gov/pmc/articles/PMC2920088/

[568] D Lukashev, B Klebanov. Cutting edge: Hypoxia-inducible factor 1alpha and its activation- inducible short isoform I.1 negatively regulate functions of CD4+ and CD8+ T lymphocytes. J Immun. Oct 15 2006. 177 (8). 4962 – 4965. DOI: https://doi.org/10.4049/jimmunol.177.8.4962 https://www.jimmunol.org/content/177/8/4962

[569] A Sant, A McMichael. Revealing the role of CD-4+ T cells in viral immunity. J Exp Med. Jul 30 2012. 209 (8). https://dx.doi.org/10.1084%2Fjem.20121517 https://www.ncbi.nlm.nih.gov/pmc/articles/PMC3420330/

[570] B Borovoy, C Huber, Maria Crisler. Masks, false safety and real dangers, Part 2: Microbial challenges from masks. Oct 2020. https://PDMJ.org

[571] J Lan, Z Song, et al. Research letter: Skin damage among health care workers managing coronavirus disease-2019. Mar 9 2020. J Am Acad Dermatol. 82 (5). 1215-1216. https://www.jaad.org/article/S0190-9622(20)30392-3/pdf

[572] US Food and Drug Administration. Definition of a medical device. Section 201(h). https://www.fda.gov/media/131268/download

[573] US Food and Drug Administration. Medical device overview. https://www.fda.gov/industry/regulated-products/medical-device-overview#What%20is%20a%20medical%20device

[574] Us Food and Drug Administration. "Who can write a prescription for a medical device?" https://www.fda.gov/medical-devices/home-use-devices/frequently-asked-questions-about-home-use-devices#5

[575] E Sinkule, J Powell, et al. Evaluation of N95 respirator use with a surgical mask cover: effects on breathing resistance and inhaled carbon dioxide. [Table 4] Ann Occup Hygiene. Oct 29 2012. 57 (3). 384-398. https://doi.org/10.1093/annhyg/mes068 https://academic.oup.com/annweh/article/57/3/384/230992

[576] Z Zhaoshi. Potential risks when some special people wear masks. No. 1 Dept of Neurology, The Third Hospital of Jilin University. Apr 18 2020. https://jamanetwork.com/journals/jama/fullarticle/2764955

Masks and COVID risks

[577] C Felter, N Bussemaker. Which countries are requiring face masks? Council on Foreign Relations. Aug 4, 2020. https://www.cfr.org/in-brief/which-countries-are-requiring-face-masks

[578] B Borovoy, C Huber, M Crisler. Masks, false safety and real dangers, Part 2: Microbial challenges from masks. Primary Doctor Med J. Nov 2020. https://pdmj.org/Mask_Risks_Part2.pdf

[579] I Miller. Mask charts. Rational Ground. https://rationalground.com/mask-charts/

[580] I Miller. More mask charts. Rational Ground. https://rationalground.com/more-mask-charts/

[581] The COVID Tracking Project. Data download. The Atlantic. https://covidtracking.com/data/download

[582] https://github.com/owid/covid-19-data/tree/master/public/data

[583] H Bundgaard, J Bundgaard, et al. Effectiveness of adding a mask recommendation to other public health measures to prevent SARS-CoV-2 infection in Danish mask wearers: A randomized controlled trial. Ann Int Med. Nov 18 2020. https://doi.org/10.7326/M20-6817. https://www.acpjournals.org/doi/10.7326/M20-6817

[584] J Xiao, E Shiu, et al. Nonpharmaceutical measures for pandemic influenza in non-healthcare settings – personal protective and environmental measures. Centers for Disease Control. 26(5); 2020 May. https://wwwnc.cdc.gov/eid/article/26/5/19-0994_article

[585] T Jefferson, M Jones, et al. Physical interventions to interrupt or reduce the spread of respiratory viruses. MedRxiv. 2020 Apr 7. https://www.medrxiv.org/content/10.1101/2020.03.30.20047217v2

[586] C Huber. Masks are neither effective nor safe: A summary of the science. PDMJ.org. Dec 2020. https://pdmj.org/Mask_Risks_Part4.pdf

[587] J Brainard, N Jones, et al. Facemasks and similar barriers to prevent respiratory illness such as COVID19: A rapid systematic review. MedRxiv. 2020 Apr 1. https://www.medrxiv.org/content/10.1101/2020.04.01.20049528v1.full.pdf

[588] E Fischer, M Fischer, et al. Low-cost measurement of face mask efficacy for filtering expelled droplets during speech. Science Advances. Sep 2 2020. 6 (36). https://advances.sciencemag.org/content/6/36/eabd3083?fbclid=IwAR0TPVlflF_sUEiSdad6oM1NVQGO5w2S7WfstCIKalJ15JJaKaDMzBkD5YY

[589] N Mitchell, S Hunt. Surgical face masks in modern operating rooms – a costly and unnecessary ritual? J Hosp Inf. Jul 1991. 18 (3): 239-242. https://doi.org/10.1016/0195-6701(91)90148-2 https://www.sciencedirect.com/science/article/abs/pii/0195670191901482

[590] M Nicas, W Nazaroff, et al. Toward understanding the risk of secondary airborne infection: Emission of respirable pathogens. J Occup and Env Hygiene. Aug 2010. 143-154. https://doi.org/10.1080/15459620590918466 https://www.tandfonline.com/doi/full/10.1080/15459620590918466

[591] M Viola, B Peterson, et al. Face coverings, aerosol dispersion and mitigation of virus transmission risk. https://arxiv.org/abs/2005.10720, https://arxiv.org/ftp/arxiv/papers/2005/2005.10720.pdf

[592] S Grinshpun, H Haruta, et al. Performance of an N95 filtering facepiece particular respirator and a surgical mask during human breathing: two pathways for particle penetration. J Occup Env Hygiene. 2009; 6(10):593-603. https://www.tandfonline.com/doi/pdf/10.1080/15459620903120086

[593] N Mitchell, S Hunt. Surgical face masks in modern operating rooms – a costly and unnecessary ritual? J Hosp Inf. Jul 1991. 18 (3): 239-242. https://doi.org/10.1016/0195-6701(91)90148-2 https://www.sciencedirect.com/science/article/abs/pii/0195670191901482

[594] US Department of Labor, Occupational Safety & Health Administration. Confined or enclosed spaces and other dangerous atmospheres >> Oxygen deficient or oxygen enriched atmospheres. https://www.osha.gov/SLTC/etools/shipyard/shiprepair/confinedspace/oxygendeficient.html

[595] B Borovoy, C Huber, M Crisler. Masks, false safety and real dangers, Part 3: Hypoxia, hypercapnia and physiological effects. PDMJ. Nov 2020. https://pdmj.org/Mask_Risks_Part3.pdf

[596] A Beder, U Buyukkocak, et al. Preliminary report on surgical mask induced deoxygenation during major surgery. Neurocirugia 2008. 19. 121-126. http://scielo.isciii.es/pdf/neuro/v19n2/3.pdf

[597] D Lukashev, B Klebanov. Cutting edge: Hypoxia-inducible factor 1alpha and its activation- inducible short isoform I.1 negatively regulate functions of CD4+ and CD8+ T lymphocytes. J Immun. Oct 15 2006. 177 (8). 4962 – 4965. DOI: https://doi.org/10.4049/jimmunol.177.8.4962 https://www.jimmunol.org/content/177/8/4962

[598] A Sant, A McMichael. Revealing the role of CD-4+ T cells in viral immunity. J Exp Med. Jul 30 2012. 209 (8).
https://dx.doi.org/10.1084%2Fjem.20121517
https://www.ncbi.nlm.nih.gov/pmc/articles/PMC3420330/

[599] R Zhang, H Su, et al. MiRNA let-7b promotes the development of hypoxic pulmonary hypertension by targeting ACE2. Am J Physiol Lung Cell Mol Physiol. Mar 2019. 1; 316 (3): L547-L557. doi: 10.1152/ajplung.00387.2018
https://pubmed.ncbi.nlm.nih.gov/30628484/

[600] P Verdecchia, C Cavallini et al. The pivotal link between ACE2 deficiency and SARS-CoV-2 infection. Eur J Intern Med. Jun 2020. 76: 14-20.
doi: 10.1016/j.ejim.2020.04.037
https://www.ncbi.nlm.nih.gov/pmc/articles/PMC7167588/

[601] B Borovoy, C Huber, M Crisler. Masks, false safety and real dangers, Part 3: Hypoxia, hypercapnia and physiological effects. PDMJ. Nov 2020.
https://pdmj.org/Mask_Risks_Part3.pdf

[602] T Jacobson, J Kler, et al. Direct human health risks of increased atmospheric carbon dioxide. Nat Sustain. 2019. 2 (8). 691-701.
https://www.nature.com/articles/s41893-019-0323-1

[603] B Chandrasekaran, S Fernandes. Exercise with facemask; Are we handling a devil's sword? – A physiological hypothesis. Nov 2020. 144 (110002).
doi: 10.1016/j.mehy.2020.110002
https://www.ncbi.nlm.nih.gov/pmc/articles/PMC7306735/#b0135

[604] M Joyner, D Casey. Regulation of increased blood flow (hyperemia) to muscles during exercise: a hierarchy of competing physiological needs. Physiol Rev. Apr 2015. 95 (2). 549-601. doi: 10.1152/physrev.00035.2013.
https://pubmed.ncbi.nlm.nih.gov/25834232/

605 C Kempeneers, C Seaton, et al. Ciliary functional analysis: beating a path towards standardization. Pediatr Pulmonol. Oct 2019. 54 (10). 1627-1638. https://doi.org/10.1002/ppul.24439 https://pubmed.ncbi.nlm.nih.gov/31313529/

606 S Casalino-Matsuda, N Wang, et al. Hypercapnia alters expression of immune response, nucleosome assembly and lipid metabolism genes in differentiated human bronchial epithelial cells. Sep 10 2018. Sci Rep. 13508. https://www.nature.com/articles/s41598-018-32008-x

607 A Schogler, R Muster, et al. Vitamin D represses rhinovirus replication in cystic fibrosis cells by inducing LL-37. Eur Resp J 2016. 47: 520-530. DOI: 10.1183/13993003.00665-2015 https://erj.ersjournals.com/content/47/2/520

608 C Gunville, P Mourani, et al. The role of vitamin D in the prevention and treatment of infection. Inflamm Allergy Drug Targets. Jul 2013. 12 (4): 239-245. https://www.ncbi.nlm.nih.gov/pmc/articles/PMC3756814/

609 P Ilie et al. The role of vitamin D in the prevention of coronavirus disease2019 infection and mortality. Aging Clin Exper Res. https://www.ncbi.nlm.nih.gov/pmc/articles/PMC7202265/pdf/40520_2020_Article_1570.pdf

Where my rights end

610 V Melnikov, V Divert, et al. Baseline values of cardiovascular and respiratory parameters predict response to acute hypoxia in young healthy men. Physiol Res. 2017. 66 (3). 467-479. https://pubmed.ncbi.nlm.nih.gov/28248531/

[611] T Kao, K Huang, et al. The physiological impact of wearing an N95 mask during hemodialysis as a precaution against SARS in patients with end-stage renal disease. J Formos Med Assoc. Aug 2004. 103 (8). 624-628. https://pubmed.ncbi.nlm.nih.gov/15340662/

[612] R Roberge, A Coca, et al. Physiological impact of the N95 filtering facepiece respirator on healthcare workers. Respir Care. May 2010. 55 (5). 569-577. https://pubmed.ncbi.nlm.nih.gov/20420727/

[613] A Beder, U Buyukkocak, et al. Preliminary report on surgical mask induced deoxygenation during major surgery. Neurocirugia 2008. 19. 121-126. http://scielo.isciii.es/pdf/neuro/v19n2/3.pdf

[614] J Williams, J Krah, et al. The physiological burden of prolonged PPE use on healthcare workers during long shifts. US Centers for Disease Control and Prevention. Jun 10 2020. https://blogs.cdc.gov/niosh-science-blog/2020/06/10/ppe-burden/

[615] Acid-base physiology, 4.4 Respiratory acidosis-Metabolic effects. https://www.anaesthesiamcq.com/AcidBaseBook/ab4_4.php

[616] J Mokili, F Rohwer, et al. Metagenomics and future perspectives in virus discovery. Curr Opin Virology. Feb 2012. 2 (1). 63-77. https://www.sciencedirect.com/science/article/abs/pii/S1879625711001908?via%3Dihub

[617] C Huber. Proposed mechanisms by which masks increase risk of COVID-19. PDMJ. Dec 7 2020. Winter 2020. https://pdmj.org/papers/masks_false_safety_and_real_dangers_part4/

[618] J Ioannidis. The infection fatality rate of COVID-19 inferred from seroprevalence data. Bulletin of the World Health Organization. Oct 14 2020. 2021; 99:19-33F. https://www.who.int/bulletin/volumes/99/1/20-265892/en/

[619] US Centers for Disease Control and Prevention (CDC). Sep 10 2020. https://www.cdc.gov/coronavirus/2019-ncov/hcp/planning-scenarios.html

[620] https://c19study.com/

[621] Coronavirus latest: South Africa variants found in Conn; Long Island ICU capacity at 80%. NPR. Feb 15 2021. https://www.wshu.org/post/coronavirus-latest-south-africa-variant-found-conn-long-island-icu-capacity-80#stream/0

[622] C St. Croix, B Morgan, et al. Fatiguing inspiratory muscle work causes reflex sympathetic activation in humans. J Physiol. Dec 1 2000. 529 Pt 2 (Pt 2). 493-504. doi: 10.1111/j.1469-7793.2000.00493.x. https://pubmed.ncbi.nlm.nih.gov/11101657/

[623] Blick. Your corona mask really is that gruesome. [article in German]. Sep 16, 2020. https://amp.blick.ch/wirtschaft/gebrauchte-exemplare-getestet-so-gruusig-ist-ihre-corona-maske-wirklich-id16096358.html?utm_source=twitter&utm_medium=social_user&utm_campaign=blick_amp

[624] C Kempeneers, C Seaton, et al. Ciliary functional analysis: beating a path towards standardization. Pediatr Pulmonol. Oct 2019. 54 (10). 1627-1638. https://doi.org/10.1002/ppul.24439 https://pubmed.ncbi.nlm.nih.gov/31313529/

[625] G Oberdorster, E Oberdorster, et al. Nanotoxicology: An emerging discipline evolving from studies of ultrafine particles. Environ Health Perspect. Jul 2005. 113(7): 823-839. doi: 10.1289/ehp.7339 https://www.ncbi.nlm.nih.gov/pmc/articles/PMC1257642/

[626] S Casalino-Matsuda, N Wang, et al. Hypercapnia alters expression of immune response, nucleosome assembly and lipid metabolism genes in differentiated human bronchial epithelial cells. Sci Rep. Sep 10 2018. 13508. https://www.nature.com/articles/s41598-018-32008-x

[627] D O'Croinin, et al. Sustained hypercapnic acidosis during pulmonary infection increases bacterial load and worsens lung injury. Crit Care Med. 36. 2128-2135. https://doi.org/10.1097/CCM.0b013e31817d1b59 https://pubmed.ncbi.nlm.nih.gov/18552698/

[628] E Laserna, O Sibila, et al. Hypocapnia and hypercapnia are predictors for ICU admission and mortality in hospitalized patients with community-acquired pneumonia. Chest. Nov 2012. 142 (5): 1193-1199. doi: 10.1378/chest.12-0576 https://pubmed.ncbi.nlm.nih.gov/22677348/

[629] Primary Doctor Medical Journal. https://PDMJ.org

[630] T Levy. COVID-19 How can I cure thee? Let me count the ways. Orthomolecular Medicine News Service. Jul 18 2020. http://orthomolecular.org/resources/omns/v16n37.shtml

Made in the USA
Middletown, DE
01 May 2022